The
Dartmouth
Atlas
of
Health Care

The Center for the
Evaluative Clinical Sciences

Dartmouth Medical School

AHA books are published by American Hospital Publishing, Inc., an American Hospital Association company

The views expressed in this publication are strictly those of the authors and do not necessarily represent official positions of the American Hospital Association.

Library of Congress Cataloging-in-Publication Data

Dartmouth Medical School. Center for the Evaluative Clinical Sciences.
    The Dartmouth atlas of health care / the Center for the Evaluative Clinical Sciences, Dartmouth Medical School.
        p.   cm.
    ISBN 1-55648-155-1 (hardcover)
    ISBN 1-55648-163-2 (softcover)
    1. Medical care—United States—Marketing—Maps. 2. Health facilities—United States—Statistics.   I. Title.
G1201.E5D3   1996   ⟨G&M⟩
362.1'0973'022—dc20   96-11510
                                                                                      CIP
                                                                                      MAP

Catalog no. 044100 (hardcover)
Catalog no. 044150 (softcover)

©1996 The Trustees of Dartmouth College

Printed in the USA

AHA is a service mark of the American Hospital Association used under license by American Hospital Publishing, Inc.

The Dartmouth Atlas of Health Care in the United States

John E. Wennberg, M.D., M.P.H., *Principal Investigator and Series Editor*

Megan McAndrew Cooper, M.B.A., M.S., *Editor*

and other members of the Dartmouth Atlas of Health Care Working Group

Co-investigators and Researchers
Thomas A. Bubolz, Ph.D.
Elliott S. Fisher, M.D., M.P.H.
Alan M. Gittelsohn, Ph.D.
David C. Goodman, M.D., M.S.
Jack E. Mohr
James F. Poage, Ph.D.
Sandra M. Sharp, S.M.
Jonathan Skinner, Ph.D.
Thérèse A. Stukel, Ph.D.

Administration, Data Production, and Technical Support
Nancy E. Cloud
Jiaqi Gong, M.S.
Kristen K. Patterson

The research to create the Dartmouth Atlas of Health Care
was made possible by a grant from

The Robert Wood Johnson Foundation

The Center for the Evaluative Clinical Sciences
Dartmouth Medical School
Hanover, New Hampshire 03756
(603) 650-1820
http://www.dartmouth.edu/~atlas/

Published in cooperation with The Center for Health Care Leadership
of the American Hospital Association

American Hospital Publishing, Inc.
Chicago, Illinois

Table of Contents

Maps

Figures

Introduction

Geographic Variations in Health Care

Health services researchers have long been aware of large variations in the use of medical care among communities and regions. In the 1930s, the British pediatrician J. Allison Glover observed that the rates of surgical removal of the tonsils in British schoolchildren varied widely, depending on the district in which the students lived and the school health doctors who examined them. In some school districts, more than 50% of children had tonsillectomies, while in others, less than 10% did. In the 1970s, studies of variation among local hospital market areas in Vermont and Maine revealed wide variations in the per capita numbers of hospital beds, employees, and physicians and noted the associations between supply of resources and use of care: more beds meant greater rates of hospitalization, and more surgeons meant more surgery. In the 1980s, a series of studies of Boston and New Haven, Connecticut (see box), extended insights into the variation phenomenon, demonstrating once again that in health care markets, geography is destiny: the care one receives depends in large part on the supply of resources available in the place where one lives – and on the practice patterns of local physicians.

The existence of variation raises a number of important issues. Foremost is the question "Which rate is right?" Which pattern of resource allocation, and which pattern of utilization, is "correct?" The study of practice variations reveals how complex this question really is. In the case of variations in rates of individual procedures, such as tonsillectomy and hysterectomy, the explanation is *not* that patients in areas with low procedure rates are going without treatment; they are, instead, being treated differently, often with more conservative medical management. Learning which rate is right requires learning what informed patients want. The right rate must be the one that reflects the choices of patients who have been adequately informed and empowered to choose among the available options.

In the case of variations in the supply of health care resources, such as the numbers of hospital beds and physicians, the question "Which rate is right?" needs to be framed in another way: What is the impact on population health of variations in resource allocation? Is more better? And if not, how much could be reallocated to

A Case Study of Variation: Boston and New Haven

The Boston, Massachusetts, and New Haven, Connecticut, hospital service areas have provided an excellent small-scale laboratory for studying variations in medical resource allocation and utilization. Both communities are similar in factors that determine the need for and access to health care, such as age, race, and income levels. Both are served by prestigious medical centers. Yet residents of the two communities are treated in very different ways, both in terms of overall health care utilization and in terms of the kinds of treatment they receive for specific conditions.

In 1989, the residents of the Boston hospital service area used more than 4.3 hospital beds for every thousand residents, compared with fewer than 2.3 beds for every thousand residents of the New Haven hospital service area. Bostonians were much more likely to be hospitalized for virtually all acute and chronic medical conditions. Most of the extra beds in Boston were used for the hospitalization of patients with such common conditions as pneumonia, heart failure, and gastroenteritis; patients with these problems who lived in the New Haven hospital service area were more likely to be treated outside of the hospital.

The reasons for the differences in the number of beds per resident included greater competition between hospitals (there were 11 acute care hospitals in Boston and only two in New Haven), the needs of academic medical centers (there were three medi-cal schools in Boston and one in New Haven), and the needs of religious communities for their own hospitals (there were four hospitals affiliated with religious groups in Boston and one in New Haven). Whatever the causes, the variations in the availability and use of hospital care resulted in substantial differences in health care spending. In 1989, the per capita expenditure for acute hospital care was $1,524 for Bostonians; for residents of New Haven, it was $777. Had the per capita rates of hospitalization and reimbursements in Boston and neighboring Brookline been the same as those in New Haven, Boston would have needed 1,529 fewer hospital beds, and expenditures for hospital care *for Bostonians alone* would have been reduced by half a billion dollars in 1989.

Patterns of surgical care, however, were much more idiosyncratic. Rates of some procedures were higher in Boston; rates of other kinds of surgery were higher in New Haven. In the 1980s, the rates for coronary artery bypass grafting surgery and for hysterectomy, per thousand Medicare enrollees, were much higher for residents of the New Haven hospital service area; Bostonians, on the other hand, were much more likely to undergo hip and knee replacement surgery. This does not mean that patients in areas with low surgical rates were necessarily underserved; they were simply cared for differently. Boston residents with coronary artery disease were more likely to be treated with medications or angioplasty than residents of New Haven. ■

other, more effective uses by reducing resources and their utilization to the level of more conservative communities?

Another important issue raised by geographic variation concerns fairness. Variation studies provide good evidence that populations in low cost regions are not sicker or in greater medical need than those in high cost regions. Costs are higher, not because better health is being achieved, but because the local health care systems have greater capacity, or because the price of medical care in these communities is higher. A system that rewards high cost areas by continuing to pay their higher costs is by definition economically punishing areas that have fewer resources, use them more efficiently, and are reimbursed less. Is it fair for citizens living in regions with low per capita health care costs to subsidize the greater (and more costly) use of care by people living in high resource and high utilization regions?

The Geography of Health Care in the United States

The first task in preparing this Atlas was to establish the geographic boundaries of naturally occurring health care markets in the United States. Based on a study of where Medicare patients were hospitalized, 3,436 geographic hospital service areas were defined. The hospital service areas were then grouped into 306 hospital referral regions on the basis of where Medicare patients were hospitalized for major cardio-vascular surgical procedures and neurosurgery, markers for regionalization. Part One of the Atlas describes how this was done, and contains a series of maps that detail each hospital referral region in the United States. One important finding was that most hospital service areas and hospital referral regions, as defined by where patients actually receive their care, correspond poorly to political configurations, such as counties, which have traditionally been used to measure health care resources and utilization.

Acute Care Hospital Resources and Expenditures

Part Two focuses on the acute care hospital capacity in each hospital referral region. After adjusting for differences in the age, sex, and race of resident populations, there were greater than twofold differences in the numbers of hospital beds per thousand residents of hospital referral regions in the United States. For example, in 1993, Honolulu had 2.2 beds per thousand residents and Seattle had 2.4. But Chicago had 4.6 beds per thousand residents and New Orleans had 5.2. The differences in hospital personnel and expenditures were of similar magnitude.

Hospital Capacity, Utilization, and Outcomes

Part Three of the Atlas provides a framework for understanding the implications of geographic variations in hospital resources, the utilization and costs of care, and the impact of these variations for one health outcome, population mortality. Variations in hospital utilization cannot be explained by differences in the underlying rates of illness; rather, they reflect two distinctive aspects of our health care system: inequal-ity in hospital capacity, and the implicit assumption in some areas that more aggressive intervention – diagnosis, hospitalization, and treatment – is better.

The Medicare Program

Part Four of the Atlas reports on federal spending for the Medicare program in each of the 306 hospital referral regions during 1993. There were important differences between regions. Total Medicare reimbursements in the Minneapolis region were about $2,800 per enrollee; in the Miami region, they were $6,400, more than twice as high. Reimbursements for inpatient care, outpatient care, physicians' services, and home health care also exhibited substantial variations; for example, home health care reimbursements in Rochester, Minnesota, were $46 per enrollee; in Chattanooga, Tennessee, they were $1,177, about 25 times higher.

The differences in Medicare's per enrollee reimbursements raise important issues concerning geographic equity and have important implications for the Medicare program.

The Physician Workforce

Since the early 1960s, the numbers of medical schools and residency training positions in the United States have increased dramatically, and the physician supply has increased correspondingly – from about 200,000 physicians in active practice in 1970 to over 450,000 in 1993, an 80% per capita increase. Part Five provides detailed information about the geographic distribution of the physician workforce in 1993. The supply of physicians varied by a factor of three, from fewer than 100 physicians per hundred thousand residents of some hospital referral regions to more than 300 in others. The variation was greater among the individual specialties, and greatest among psychiatrists, where the supply varied from a low of 2.5 per hundred thousand residents to a high of 43.9.

The Diagnosis and Surgical Treatment of Common Medical Conditions

Part Six of the Atlas documents wide variation in the use of diagnostic and surgical procedures for people with coronary artery disease, prostate cancer, breast cancer, and back pain. The magnitude of the geographic variation is remarkable. There was a fourfold variation in per capita rates of coronary artery bypass surgery in 1992-93 among Medicare enrollees. There was an eightfold variation in rates of radical prostatectomy, an operation used to treat early stage prostate cancer. Variations in the use of breast sparing surgery in the treatment of breast cancer were over 33-fold.

Benchmarking the Patterns of Resource Allocation and Care

The aggregate quantities of hospital resources and physicians available for the care of residents of the United States are not determined by well-established evidence concerning the relationship between need and clinical outcomes. If more resources and care cannot be demonstrated to be better for a community's health outcomes, it may well be reasonable for patients, and in the public interest, to reduce the health care system's capacity to the levels of regions that have conservative levels of resources and utilization. Part Seven provides estimates of the number of hospital beds, personnel, and expenditures that could be reallocated to another use if the rates in more efficient regions became the standard of practice. For example, if the resources in all hospital referral regions in the United States that have greater supplies of hospital resources than Minneapolis were brought down to the level in the Minneapolis region, nearly 120,000 hospital beds would be closed, and $32.6 billion could be saved (or spent for a more effective purpose). Similar analysis is provided for physician staffing levels, leading to similar conclusions; if, for example, all hospital referral regions in the United States had per capita physician workforces no higher than the numbers employed by a well-established health maintenance organization, the number of physicians now active in the workforce, and the numbers being trained and brought into the workforce, would be profoundly affected.

Tables

Part Eight provides detailed information about each hospital referral region, including most of the variables presented in the Atlas. A more extensive database is available in machine-readable form.

Strategies and Methods

Part Nine provides details of the methods used in the Atlas and an explanation of the distribution graphs and the measure of association – the R^2 statistic – used in the Atlas.

About Rates in the Atlas

In order to make comparisons easier, all rates in the Atlas are expressed in terms that result in at least one digit to the left of the decimal point (e.g., 1.6 cardiologists per hundred thousand residents, 3.9 hospital beds per thousand residents). In order to achieve this result, different denominators were used in calculating rates.

The levels of supply of hospital beds and hospital full time equivalent employees are expressed as beds and employees per thousand residents of the hospital referral region, based on American Hospital Association and Medicare data.

Expenditures and reimbursements are expressed as dollars per capita, or per resident of the hospital referral region, based on Medicare claims data and census calculations.

The numbers of physicians providing services to residents of hospital referral regions are expressed as physicians per hundred thousand residents, based on American Medical Association and American Osteopathic Association data and census calculations.

The numbers of surgical and diagnostic procedures performed are expressed as procedures per thousand Medicare enrollees in the hospital referral region, or as procedures per thousand male or female Medicare enrollees in the region – for procedures like prostatectomy or mammography that apply only to one sex – based on Medicare claims data.

Patient day rates are expressed as total inpatient days per thousand Medicare enrollees.

Making Fair Comparisons Between Regions

Some areas of the country have greater needs for health care services and resources than others; for example, in some communities in Florida, as many as 60% of residents are over 65, while other areas – including some with large college populations, or ski resorts – have much larger proportions of younger people. To ensure fair comparisons between regions, all rates in the Atlas have been adjusted to remove the differences that might be due to the age and sex composition of regional populations. This adjustment avoids identifying some regions as having high rates of utilization simply because of their larger proportions of elderly residents. When data were available, rates have also been adjusted for differences in race. The methods used to adjust these rates are explained in Part Nine.

Some parts of the country, such as major urban areas, have higher costs of living than others. Such areas are likely to have higher health care expenditures because the cost of personnel, real estate, and supplies are higher, and not necessarily because they are providing more services. Adjusting for such variation provides a better measure of differences in real health care spending, not simply differences attributable to the fact that some regions are more expensive in which to live than others. To ensure fair comparisons of health care expenditures, hospital expenditure rates and Medicare reimbursement rates were adjusted to take into account regional differences in costs of living.

The methods used to adjust for age, sex, race, and price of medical care are detailed in Part Nine of the Atlas.

Communicating With Us About the Atlas

Our Atlas Home Page on the World Wide Web contains Atlas information, including a summary of Dartmouth related research and electronic copies of some hard to find references. Please send us your comments on the Atlas, particularly suggestions on how to improve it in the future. We are at http://www.dartmouth.edu/~atlas/

PART ONE

The Geography of Health Care in the United States

The Geography of Health Care in the United States

The use of health care resources in the United States is highly localized. Most Americans use the services of physicians whose practices are nearby. Physicians, in turn, are usually affiliated with hospitals that are near their practices. As a result, when patients are admitted to hospitals, the admission generally takes place within a relatively short distance of where the patient lives. This is true across the United States. Although the distances from homes to hospitals vary with geography – people who live in rural areas travel farther than those who live in cities – in general most patients are admitted to a hospital close to where they live which provides an appropriate level of care.

The Medicare program maintains exhaustive records of hospitalizations, which makes it possible to define the patterns of use of hospital care. When Medicare enrollees are admitted to hospitals, the program's records identify both the patients' places of residence (by ZIP Code) and the hospitals where the admissions took place (by a unique numerical identifier). These files provide a reliable basis for determining the geographic pattern of health care use, because research shows that the migration patterns of patients in the Medicare program are similar to those for younger patients.

Medicare records of hospitalizations were used to define 3,436 geographically distinct hospital service areas in the United States. In each hospital service area, most of the care received by Medicare patients is provided in hospitals within the area. Based on the patterns of care for major cardiovascular surgery and neurosurgery, hospital service areas were aggregated into 306 hospital referral regions; this Atlas reports on patterns of care in these hospital referral regions.

How Hospital Service Areas Were Defined

Hospital service areas were defined through a three-step process. First, all acute care hospitals in the 50 states and the District of Columbia were identified from the American Hospital Association and Medicare provider files and assigned to the town or city in which they were located. The name of the town or city was used as the name of the hospital service area, even though the area might have extended well beyond the political boundary of the town. For example, the Mt. Ascutney Hospital is in Windsor, Vermont. The area is called the Windsor hospital service area, even though the area serves several other communities.

In the second step, all 1992 and 1993 Medicare hospitalization records for each hospital were analyzed to ascertain the ZIP Code of each of its patients. When a town or city had more than one hospital, the counts were added together. Using a plurality rule, each ZIP Code was assigned on a provisional basis to the town containing the hospitals most often used by local residents.

The analysis of the patterns of use of care by Medicare patients led to the provisional assignment of five post office ZIP Codes to the Windsor hospital service area.

ZIP Code	Community Name	1990 Population	% of Medicare Discharges to Mt. Ascutney Hospital
05037	Brownsville	415	52.8
05048	Hartland	1,730	46.8
05053	Pomfret	245	52.6
05062	Reading	614	36.8
05089	Windsor	5,406	63.2

The third step involved the visual examination of the ZIP Codes using a computer-generated map to make sure that the ZIP Codes included in the hospital service areas were contiguous. In the case of the Windsor area, inspection of the map led to the reassignment of Pomfret to the Lebanon hospital service area. In the final determination, the Windsor hospital service area contained four communities and a total population of 8,165.

Details about the method of constructing hospital service areas are given in Part Nine.

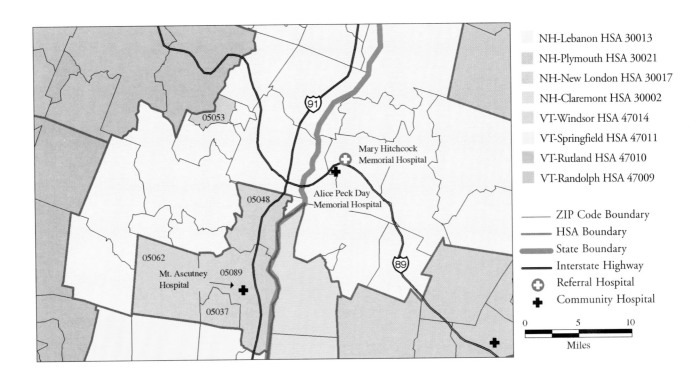

NH-Lebanon HSA 30013
NH-Plymouth HSA 30021
NH-New London HSA 30017
NH-Claremont HSA 30002
VT-Windsor HSA 47014
VT-Springfield HSA 47011
VT-Rutland HSA 47010
VT-Randolph HSA 47009

—— ZIP Code Boundary
—— HSA Boundary
—— State Boundary
—— Interstate Highway
Referral Hospital
Community Hospital

0   5   10
Miles

Map 1.1. ZIP Codes Assigned to the Windsor, Vermont, Hospital Service Area

The analysis of the pattern of use of hospitals revealed that Medicare enrollees living in the five ZIP Code areas in light blue most often used the Mt. Ascutney Hospital in Windsor, Vermont. To maintain geographic continuity of hospital service areas, the Pomfret ZIP Code 05053 was reassigned to the Lebanon hospital service area. The Windsor hospital service area contained four communities, with a 1990 census of 8,165. During 1992-93, there were 679 hospitalizations among the Medicare population; 394 (58%) were to Mt. Ascutney Hospital, 131 to the Mary Hitchcock Memorial Hospital, and 154 to other hospitals.

Hospital Service Areas in the United States

The documentation of the patterns of use of hospitals according to Medicare enrollee ZIP Codes during 1992-93 led to the aggregation of approximately 42,000 ZIP Codes into 3,436 hospital service areas. In each area, more Medicare patients were hospitalized locally than in any other single hospital service area. The propensity of patients to use local hospitals is measured by the localization index, which is the percentage of all residents' hospitalizations that occur in local hospitals (the number of local hospitalizations of residents divided by all hospitalizations of residents). This index varied from a low of 17.9% to over 94%. More than 85% of Americans lived in hospital service areas where the majority of Medicare hospitalizations occurred locally. More than 51% lived in areas where the localization index exceeded 70%.

In 1993, most Americans lived in hospital service areas with three or fewer local hospitals. Eighty-two percent, or 2,830, of all hospital service areas, which comprised 39% of the population in 1990, had only one hospital. Four hundred twenty-eight hospital service areas, which comprised 23% of the United States population, had either two or three hospitals. One hundred seventy-eight, or less than 6% of hospital service areas, had four or more local hospitals and comprised about 37% of the population of the United States.

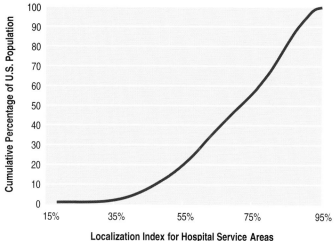

Figure 1.1. Cumulative Percentage of Population of the United States According to the Hospital Service Area Localization Index (1992-93)

The localization index is the proportion of all hospitalizations for area residents that occur in a hospital or hospitals within the area. The figure shows the localization index for Medicare patients in 3,436 hospital service areas, according to the cumulative proportion of the population living in the region. Most of the population lived in regions where more than 50% of hospitalizations occurred locally.

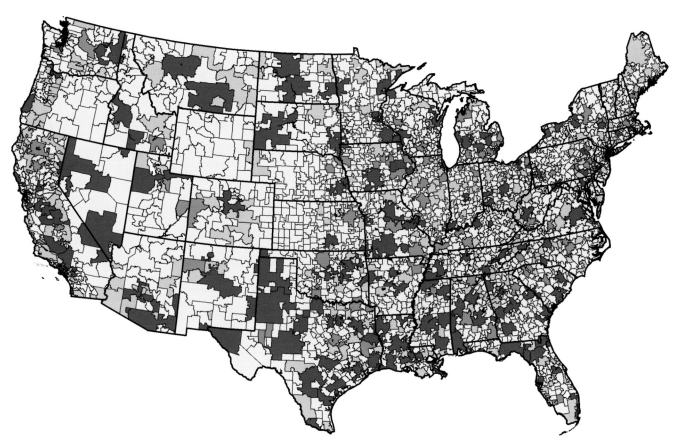

Map 1.2. Hospital Service Areas According to the Number of Acute Care Hospitals

Thirty-nine percent of the population of the United States lived in areas with one hospital (buff); 15% lived in areas with two hospitals (light orange); 8.4% lived in areas with three hospitals (bright orange); and 37% of the population lived in areas with four or more hospitals within the hospital service area (red).

Count of Acute Care Hospitals
by Hospital Service Area (1993)

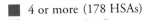

■ 4 or more	(178 HSAs)
■ 3	(106)
▨ 2	(322)
□ 1	(2,830)
▨ Not Populated	

Population Size in Hospital Service Areas

In 1993, most of the nation's 3,436 hospital service areas had relatively small populations; 92% had fewer than 180,000 residents. The 1990 census reported that about 50% of the population of the United States lived in such regions. Only 32% of Americans lived in hospital service areas with populations above 360,000 in 1990. This has important implications for health care markets, because communities with populations of fewer than 360,000 are probably too small to support independent, competing health plans. Market research suggests that in such communities, hospital resources must be shared among health plans in order to achieve efficiency. A population of 180,000 could support three plans which provided primary care and some basic specialty services but shared inpatient facilities.

More than 52% of the nation's 3,436 hospital service areas had fewer than 30,000 residents; these areas comprised about 10% of the population of the United States. In these areas, the population may be too small to support competition between even primary care physician networks.

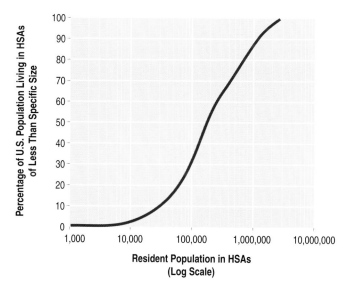

Figure 1.2. Cumulative Percentage of Population of the United States According to the Population Size of Hospital Service Areas (1990 Census)

Most Americans lived in hospital service areas with fewer than 360,000 residents, the minimum size required to support three independent health plans.

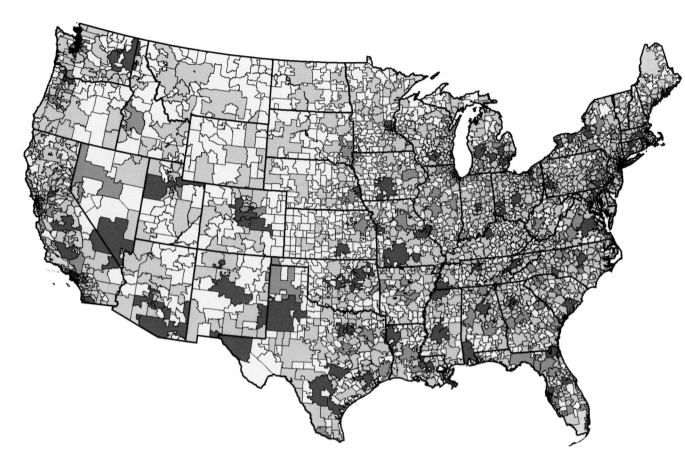

Map 1.3. Hospital Service Areas According to Population Size

According to the 1990 census, about 10% of the population of the United States lived in areas with populations of fewer than 30,000; about 50% lived in areas with fewer than 180,000 residents. Only 32% of Americans lived in hospital service areas with populations greater than 360,000.

Population of Hospital Service Areas

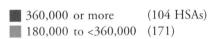

■	360,000 or more	(104 HSAs)
■	180,000 to <360,000	(171)
▨	30,000 to <180,000	(1,344)
□	866 to <30,000	(1,817)
▨	Not Populated	

How Hospital Referral Regions Were Defined

Hospital service areas make clear the patterns of use of local hospitals. A significant proportion of care, however, is provided by referral hospitals that serve a larger region. Hospital referral regions were defined in this Atlas by documenting where patients were referred for major cardiovascular surgical procedures and for neurosurgery. Each hospital service area was examined to determine where most of its residents went for these services. The result was the aggregation of the 3,436 hospital service areas into 306 hospital referral regions. Each hospital referral region had at least one city where both major cardiovascular surgical procedures and neurosurgery were performed. Maps were used to make sure that the small number of "orphan" hospital service areas – those surrounded by hospital service areas allocated to a different hospital referral region – were reassigned, in almost all cases, to ensure geographic contiguity. Hospital referral regions were pooled with neighbors if their populations were less than 120,000 or if less than 65% of their residents' hospitalizations occurred within the region.

Hospital referral regions were named for the hospital service area containing the referral hospital or hospitals most often used by residents of the region. The regions sometimes cross state boundaries. The Evansville, Indiana, hospital referral region (Map 1.4) provides an example of a region that is located in three states: Illinois, Indiana, and Kentucky. In this region, three hospitals provided cardiovascular surgery services. Two were in Evansville; a third hospital, in Vincennes, Indiana, also provided cardiovascular surgery, but in the years of this study residents of the Vincennes area used cardiovascular and neurosurgery procedures provided in Evansville more frequently than those in Vincennes, resulting in the assignment of the Vincennes hospital service area to the Evansville hospital referral region.

Map 1.4 also provides an example of a region with a population too small to meet the minimum criterion for designation as a hospital referral region. The Madisonville, Kentucky, hospital service area met the criterion as a hospital referral region on the basis of the plurality rule, but its population was less than 57,000. The area was assigned to the Paducah, Kentucky, hospital referral region because hospitals in Paducah were the second most commonly used place of care for cardiovascular and neurosurgical procedures.

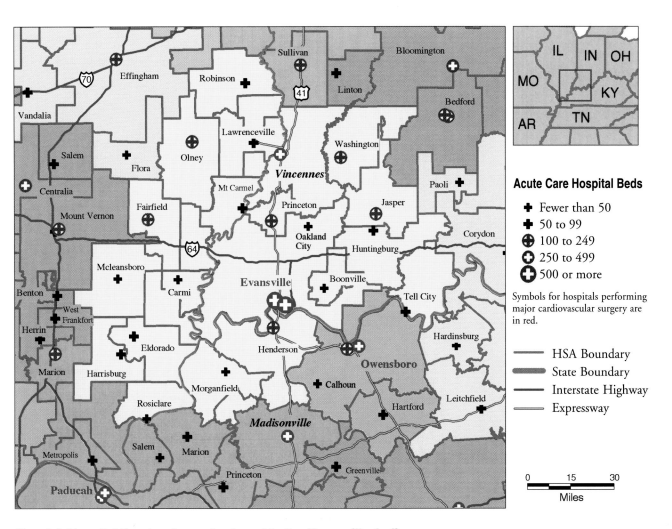

Map 1.4. Hospital Service Areas Assigned to the Evansville, Indiana, Hospital Referral Region

Hospital referral regions are named for the hospital service area containing the referral hospital or hospitals most often used by residents of the region. Hospital referral regions overlap state boundaries in every state except Alaska and Hawaii. The Evansvillle, Indiana, hospital referral region is in parts of three states: Illinois, Indiana, and Kentucky.

The Hospital Referral Regions in the United States

Among the 306 hospital referral regions in the United States, the localization index ranged from 66% to over 97%; the median was 87.5%. Ninety-one percent of Americans lived in hospital referral regions in which more than 80% of hospitalizations occurred locally.

The hospital referral regions' populations ranged from 121,666, in Bend, Oregon, to 8,891,233 in Los Angeles. One hundred fifty-one regions, or 49%, comprising 17% of the population of the United States, had populations of fewer than 500,000. Seventy-four hospital referral regions, or 24%, comprising 60% of the population, had more than one million residents, according to the 1990 census.

The number of hospitals providing major cardiovascular surgery within the hospital referral region ranged from one (in most regions) to 37 in Los Angeles. One hundred twenty-two, or 40%, of the 306 hospital referral regions had only one hospital that performed major cardiovascular surgery. One hundred fourteen, or 37%, had two or three hospitals providing these services; 70, or 23%, had four or more.

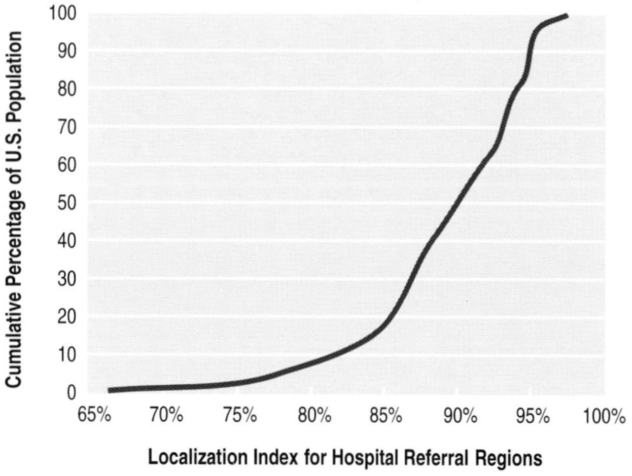

Figure 1.3. Cumulative Percentage of Population of the United States According to the Hospital Referral Region Localization Index (1992-93)

The localization index is the proportion of all hospitalizations for area residents that occurred in a hospital or hospitals within the region. Ninety-one percent of Americans lived in regions in which more than 80% of hospitalizations occurred locally.

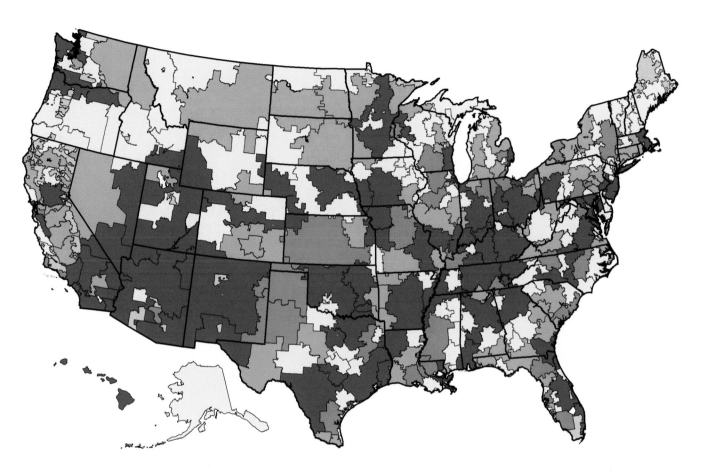

Map 1.5. Hospital Referral Regions According to the Number of Hospitals Performing Major Cardiovascular Surgery

Seventeen percent of the population of the United States lived in hospital referral regions with one hospital offering major cardiovascular surgery (buff), 18% in areas with two (light orange), 11% in regions with three (bright orange), and 54% in regions with four or more (red).

Number of Hospitals Performing Major Cardiovascular Surgery
by Hospital Referral Region (1993)

- ◼ 4 or more (70 HRRs)
- ◼ 3   (36)
- ◻ 2   (78)
- ◻ 1   (122)
- ◻ Not Populated

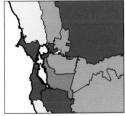

San Francisco

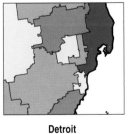

Chicago

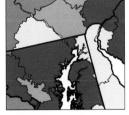

Detroit

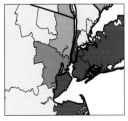

Washington-Baltimore

New York

Maps of Hospital Referral Regions in the United States

The maps on the following pages outline the boundaries of the hospital referral regions. Although in some regions more than one city provided referral care, each hospital referral region was named for the city where most patients receiving major cardiovascular surgical procedures and neurosurgery were referred for care.

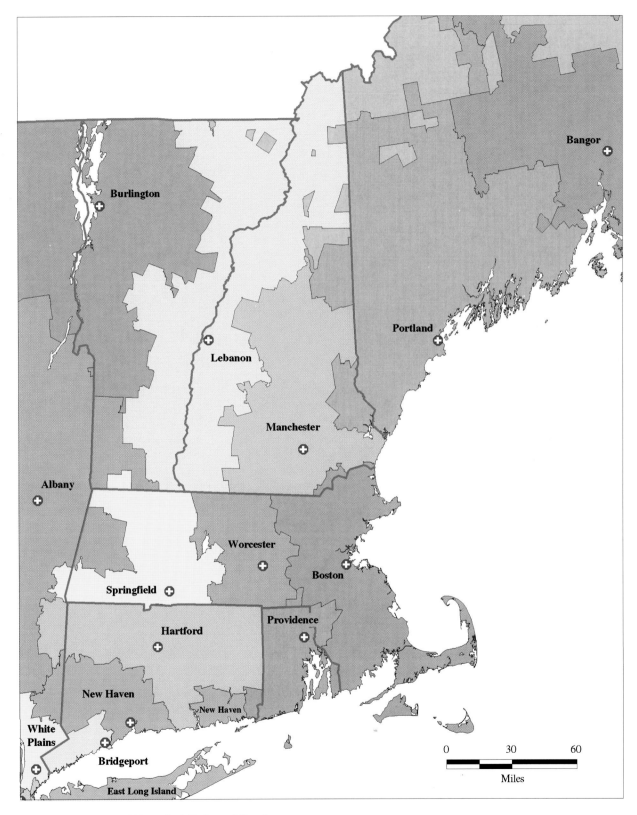

Map 1.6. New England Hospital Referral Regions

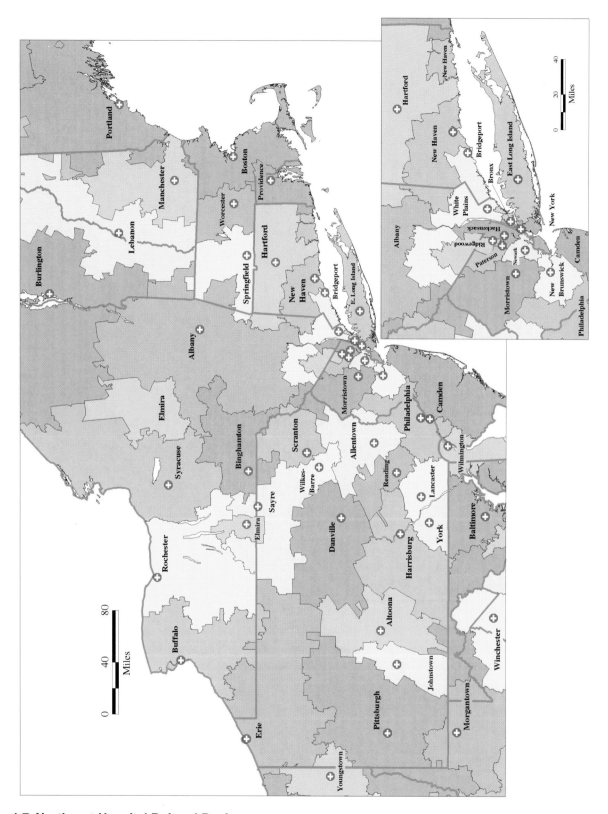

Map 1.7. Northeast Hospital Referral Regions

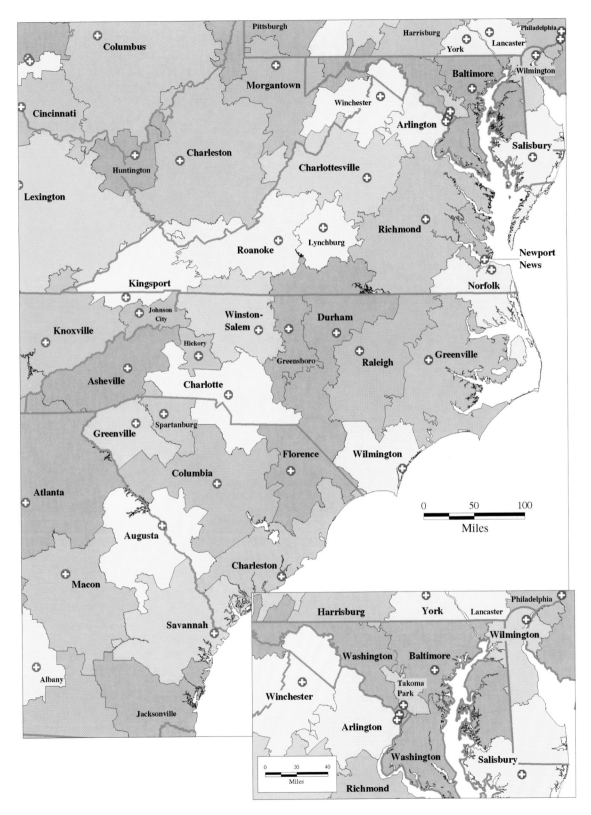

Map 1.8. South Atlantic Hospital Referral Regions

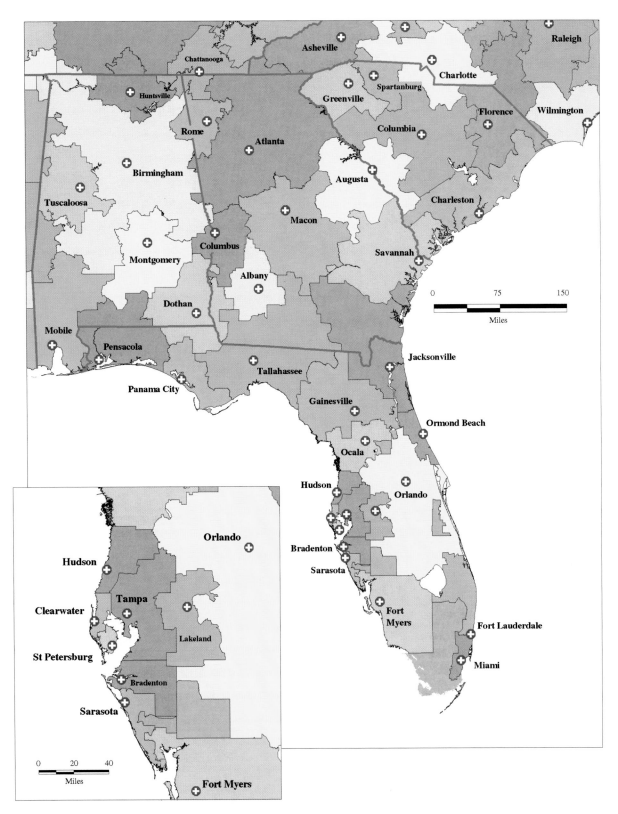

Map 1.9. Southeast Hospital Referral Regions

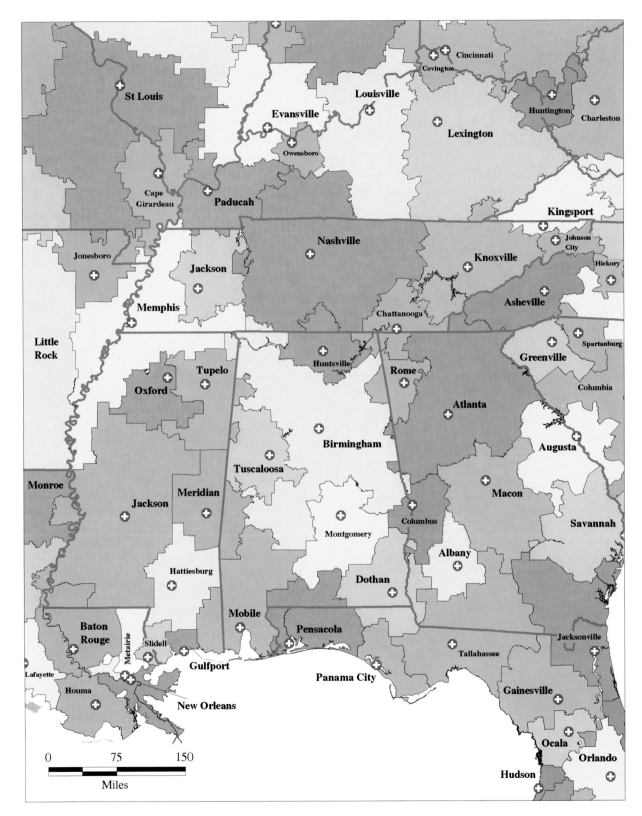

Map 1.10. South Central Hospital Referral Regions

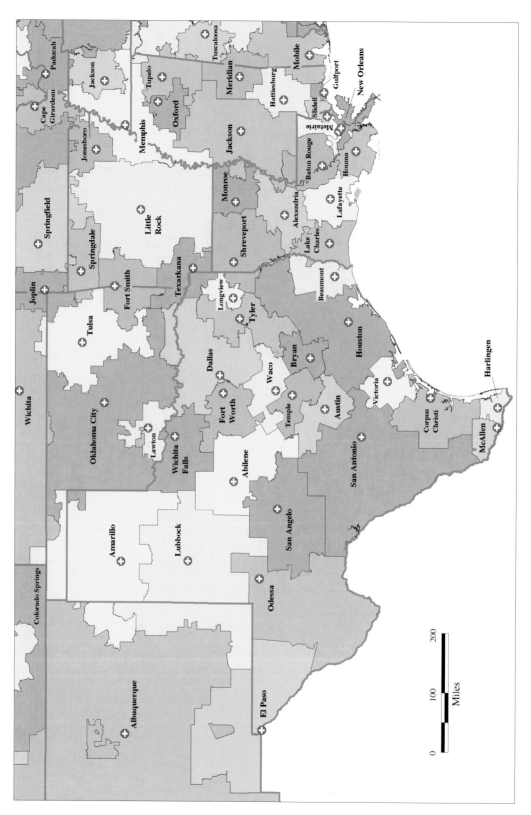

Map 1.11. Southwest Hospital Referral Regions

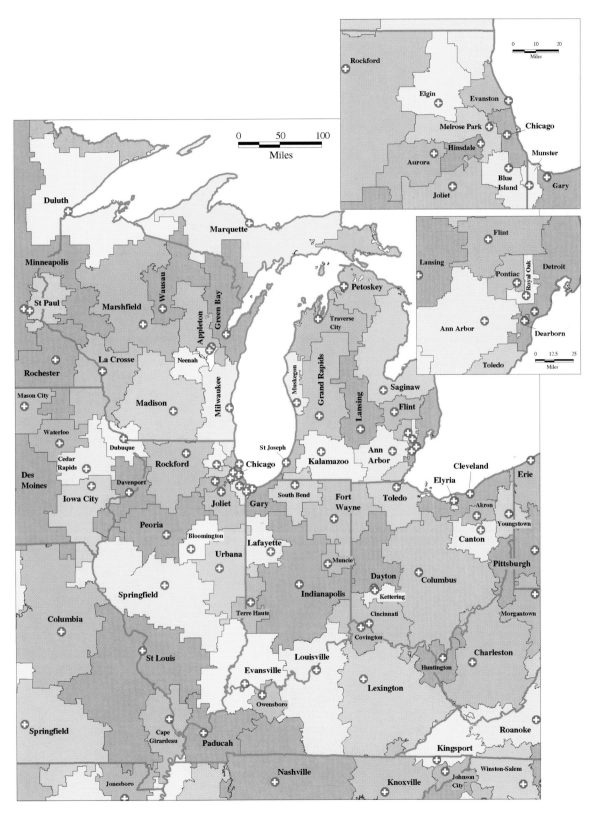

Map 1.12. Great Lakes Hospital Referral Regions

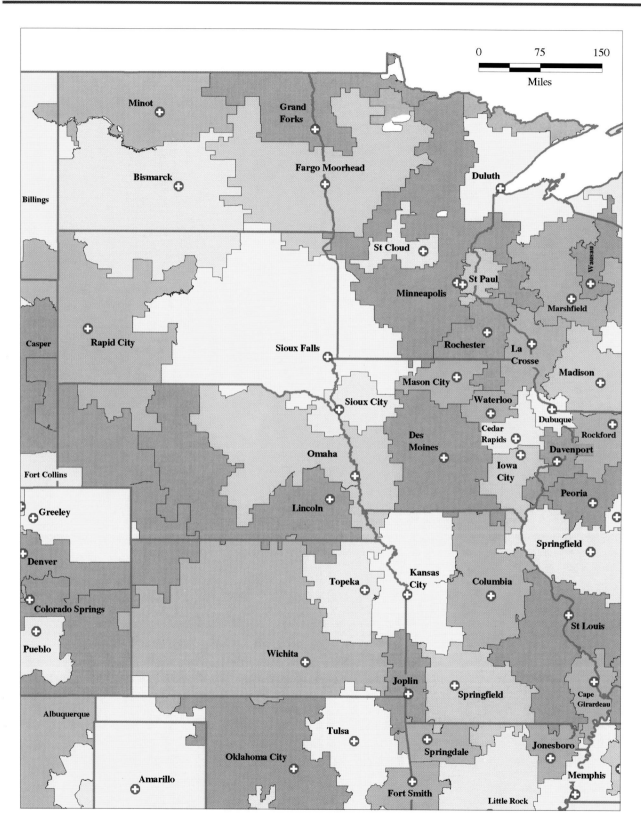

Map 1.13. Upper Midwest Hospital Referral Regions

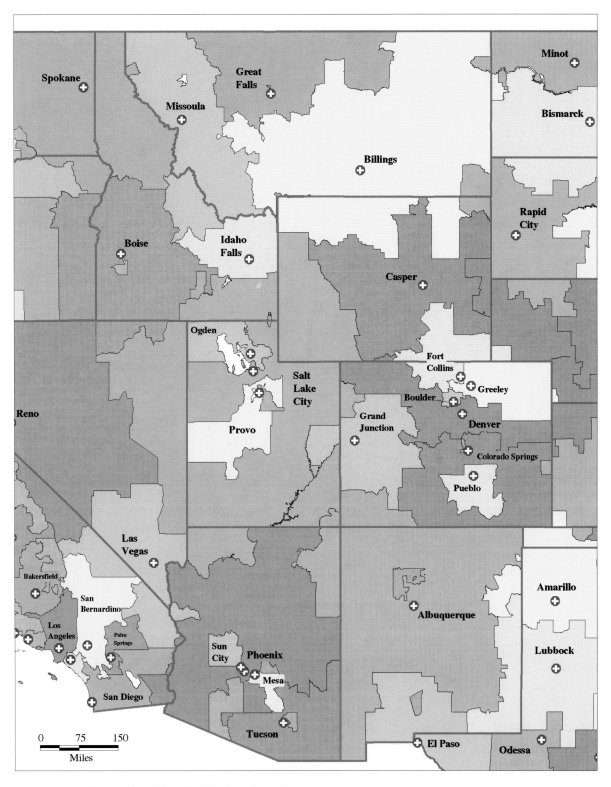

Map 1.14. Rocky Mountains Hospital Referral Regions

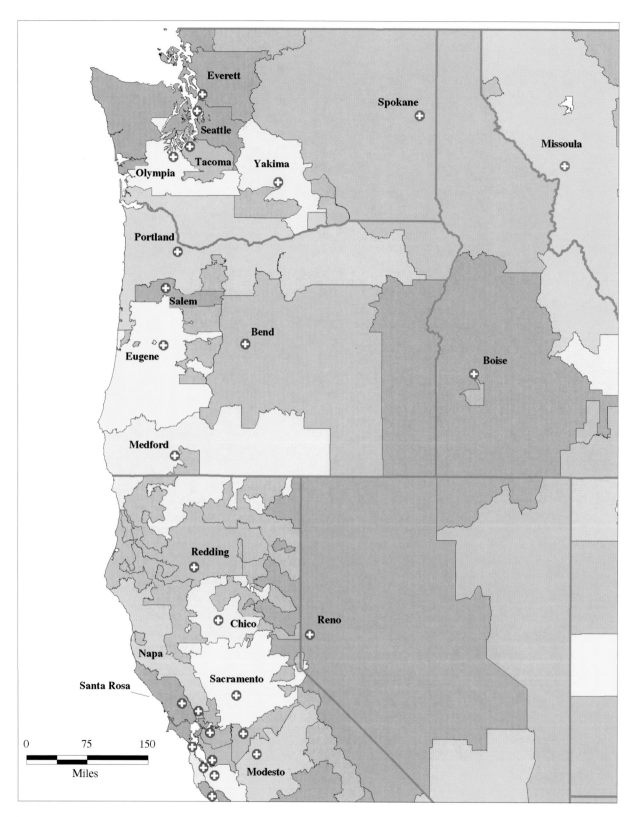

Map 1.15. Pacific Northwest Hospital Referral Regions

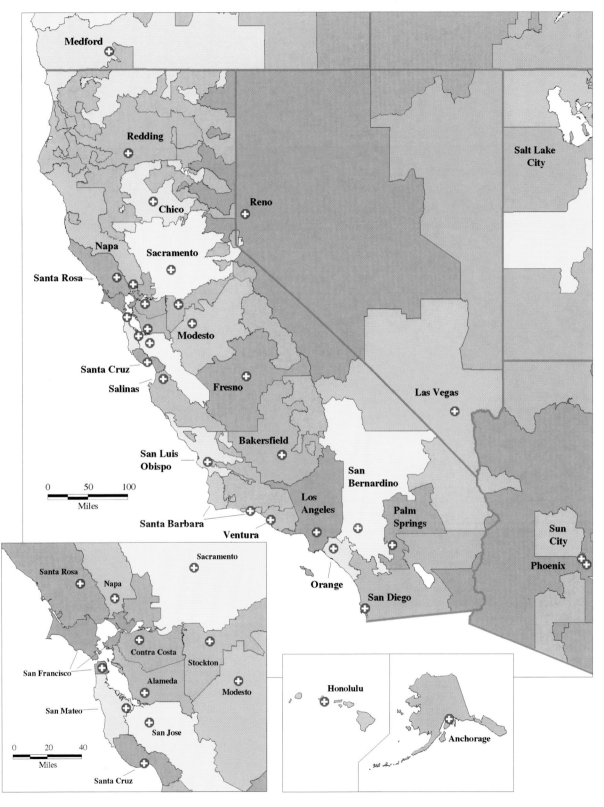

Map 1.16. Pacific Coast Hospital Referral Regions

Acute Care Hospital Resources and Expenditures

This section provides measures of the allocation of hospital resources to the populations living in the nation's 306 hospital referral regions. Data from the American Hospital Association and the Medicare Program were used to estimate the numbers of staffed hospital beds, full time equivalent hospital employees, registered nurses employed in acute care hospitals, and hospital expenditures allocated to care for the population of each region. The population count is from the 1990 United States census.

The estimates for resource allocations presented in the Atlas have been adjusted for differences in age, sex, and, in the case of expenditures, regional differences in prices. The allocation method adjusts for patient migration to hospitals located outside of the hospital referral region where the patient resides. Part Nine explains how these adjustments were done.

Acute Care Hospital Beds

There were more than 827,000 acute care hospital beds in the United States in 1993, an average of 3.3 hospital beds per thousand residents. The numbers of hospital beds per thousand persons, after adjusting for differences in age and sex, varied by a factor of 2.8, from fewer than 2 beds per thousand residents in Mesa, Arizona (1.9); Santa Cruz, California (1.9); and Everett, Washington (2.0), to more than 5 in Bismarck, North Dakota (5.2); New Orleans (5.2); and Monroe, Louisiana (5.3).

Among the hospital referral regions with large populations, those with the highest numbers of hospital beds per thousand residents were the Bronx, New York (4.9); Jackson, Mississippi (4.7); Newark, New Jersey (4.7); Manhattan (4.6); and Chicago (4.6).

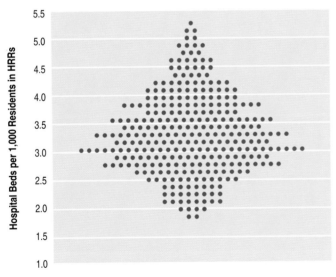

Figure 2.1. Acute Care Hospital Beds Allocated to Hospital Referral Regions (1993)

The number of hospital beds per thousand residents, after adjusting for differences in the age and sex of the local population, ranged from fewer than two to more than five. Each point represents one of the 306 hospital referral regions in the United States.

Regions with more than one million residents that had comparatively low numbers of beds per thousand residents were San Jose, California (2.1); Seattle (2.2); Arlington, Virginia (2.2); Honolulu (2.4); and New Haven, Connecticut (2.5).

The numbers of hospital beds in some cases varied strikingly between neighboring hospital referral regions. For example, the Augusta, Georgia, hospital referral region had 4.2 beds per thousand residents, but the contiguous hospital referral region in Columbia, South Carolina, had 3.2. Sioux Falls, South Dakota, had 4.2 beds per thousand, but the neighboring Minneapolis hospital referral region had only 2.8.

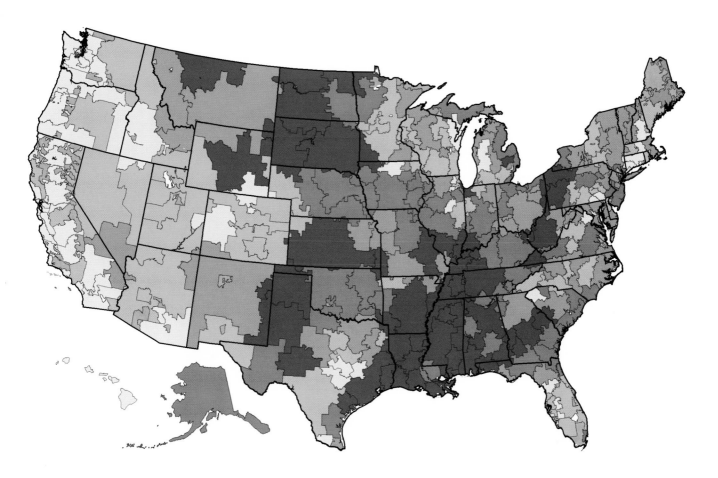

Map 2.1. Acute Care Hospital Beds

There were clear patterns of variation in the supply of hospital beds per thousand residents across the United States in 1993. The West Coast, parts of the East Coast, and some other areas had relatively few beds per thousand residents, but the Midwest, Upper Midwest, and South had high numbers of beds per thousand residents.

Acute Care Hospital Beds per 1,000 Residents

by Hospital Referral Region (1993)

- 3.96 to 5.30 (60 HRRs)
- 3.45 to <3.96 (62)
- 3.08 to <3.45 (61)
- 2.75 to <3.08 (61)
- 1.86 to <2.75 (62)
- Not Populated

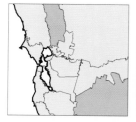

San Francisco

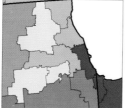

Chicago

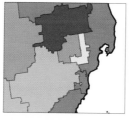

Detroit

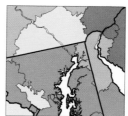

Washington-Baltimore

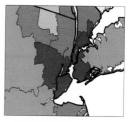

New York

Acute Care Hospital Employees

There were more than 3.56 million workers employed in acute care hospitals in the United States in 1993. The numbers of full time equivalent hospital employees per thousand residents, after adjusting for differences in population age and sex, varied by a factor of 3.3, from 8 or fewer in Mesa, Arizona (8.0); Bradenton, Florida (7.9); Santa Cruz, California (7.2); and Mason City, Iowa (6.5), to more than 21 in Chicago (21.0); New Orleans (21.2); Manhattan (22.3); Monroe, Louisiana (24.0); and the Bronx, New York (26.4).

Other hospital referral regions with high numbers of employees per thousand residents included Munster, Indiana (19.1); Newark, New Jersey (19.0); Johnstown, Pennsylvania (19.0); Detroit (18.8); and Meridian, Mississippi (18.4). Among hospital referral regions with low numbers of personnel per thousand residents were San Diego (9.8); Austin, Texas (9.0); and Clearwater, Florida (8.9).

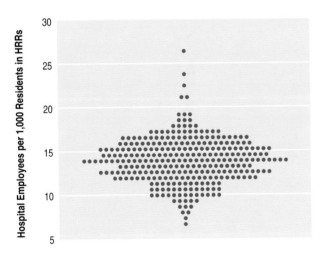

Figure 2.2. Hospital Employees Allocated to Hospital Referral Regions (1993)

The number of full time equivalent hospital employees per thousand residents, after adjusting for differences in the age and sex of the local population, ranged from 6.5 to more than 26. Each point represents one of the 306 hospital referral regions in the United States.

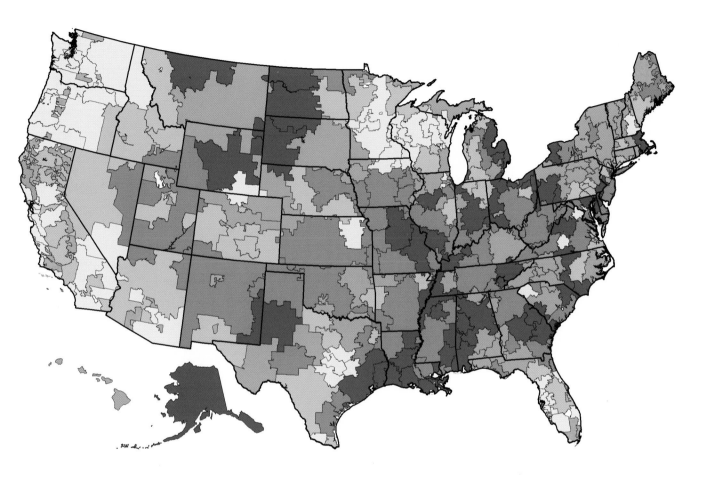

Map 2.2. Acute Care Hospital Employees

There were clear patterns of variation in the numbers of hospital employees per thousand residents in hospital referral regions across the United States in 1993. The West Coast, parts of the East Coast, and some other areas had relatively few, but the Midwest, Northeast, and South tended to have larger workforces devoted to acute care.

Hospital Employees per 1,000 Residents
by Hospital Referral Region (1993)

- ■ 15.85 to 26.42 (61 HRRs)
- ■ 14.48 to <15.85 (63)
- ■ 13.30 to <14.48 (61)
- ■ 11.93 to <13.30 (57)
- □ 6.50 to <11.93 (64)
- ■ Not Populated

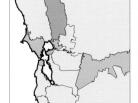

San Francisco

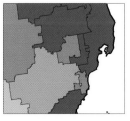

Chicago

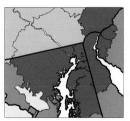

Detroit

Washington-Baltimore

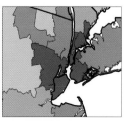

New York

Registered Nurses Employed in Acute Care Hospitals

In 1993, there were more than 872,000 full time equivalent registered nurses employed in acute care hospitals in the United States, representing about one-quarter of all hospital employees. The numbers of hospital-employed registered nurses per thousand residents, after adjusting for differences in age and sex of the local population, varied by a factor of 3.4, from fewer than 2 per thousand residents in Mason City, Iowa (1.6), and Bradenton, Florida (1.9), to 5 or more per thousand in the Bronx, New York (5.4), and Chicago (5.0).

Among hospital referral regions with high numbers of registered nurses per thousand residents were Anchorage, Alaska (4.8); Cedar Rapids, Iowa (4.7); Toledo, Ohio (4.7); Gulfport, Mississippi (4.7); Philadelphia (4.6); and Casper, Wyoming (4.6).

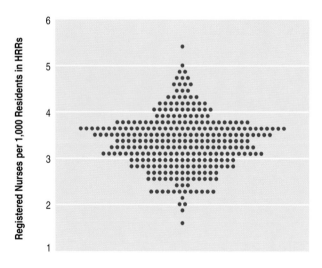

Figure 2.3. Hospital-Based Registered Nurses Allocated to Hospital Referral Regions (1993)

The acute care hospital-employed registered nurse workforce varied from 1.6 per thousand residents to 5.4. Each point represents one of the 306 hospital referral regions in the United States.

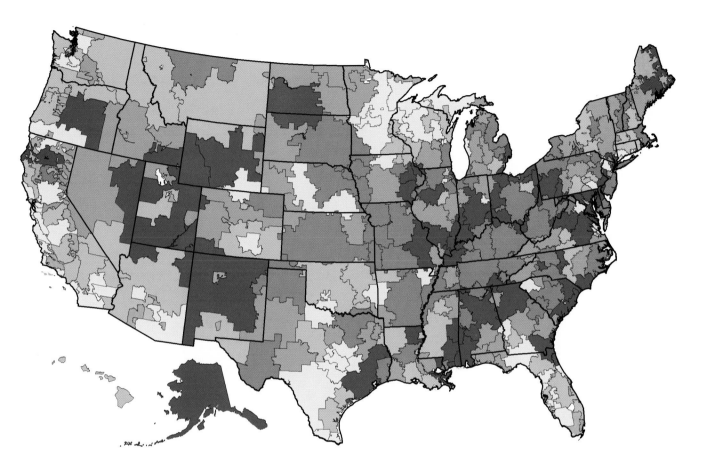

Map 2.3. Registered Nurses Employed in Acute Care Hospitals

There were more hospital-employed registered nurses per thousand residents in areas of the Midwest and West, and in parts of the East, and fewer in most of California, Minnesota, Michigan, and parts of Florida and Texas in 1993.

**Registered Nurses
per 1,000 Residents**
by Hospital Referral Region (1993)

- 3.80 to   5.43 (60 HRRs)
- 3.55 to <3.80 (63)
- 3.25 to <3.55 (61)
- 2.90 to <3.25 (59)
- 1.64 to <2.90 (63)
- Not Populated

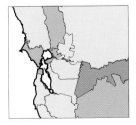

San Francisco

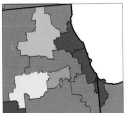

Chicago

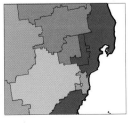

Detroit

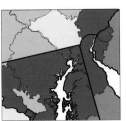

Washington-Baltimore

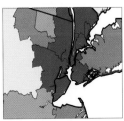

New York

Total Acute Care Hospital Expenditures

According to American Hospital Association records, the nation spent $260.9 billion on hospital care in 1993, an average of $1,049 per capita. Even after adjusting for age, sex, and regional differences in prices (see Part Nine for a description of the methods used), the per capita expenditures for hospital care varied by a factor of 2.5, from $651 or less in Mason City, Iowa ($503), and Arlington, Virginia ($651), to more than $1,600 per capita in New Orleans ($1,646) and the Bronx, New York ($1,682).

Among other hospital referral regions with high per capita expenditures for hospital care in 1993 were Chicago ($1,475), Manhattan ($1,467), Houston ($1,354), Pittsburgh ($1,315), Philadelphia ($1,295), Cincinnati ($1,278), and Detroit ($1,263).

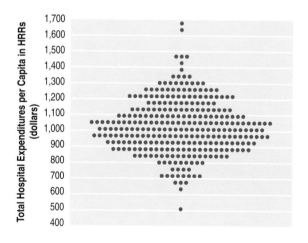

Among the hospital referral regions with low per capita expenditures were Takoma Park, Maryland ($703); Austin, Texas ($750); San Diego ($764); San Jose, California ($788); Morristown, New Jersey ($816); Orange County, California ($808); New Haven, Connecticut ($851); and Portland, Oregon ($856).

Figure 2.4. Price Adjusted Acute Care Hospital Expenditures Allocated to Hospital Referral Regions (1993)

Price adjusted per capita expenditures for inpatient and outpatient care delivered by acute care hospitals varied by a factor of more than 3, from about $500 to nearly $1,700. Each point represents one of the 306 hospital referral regions in the United States.

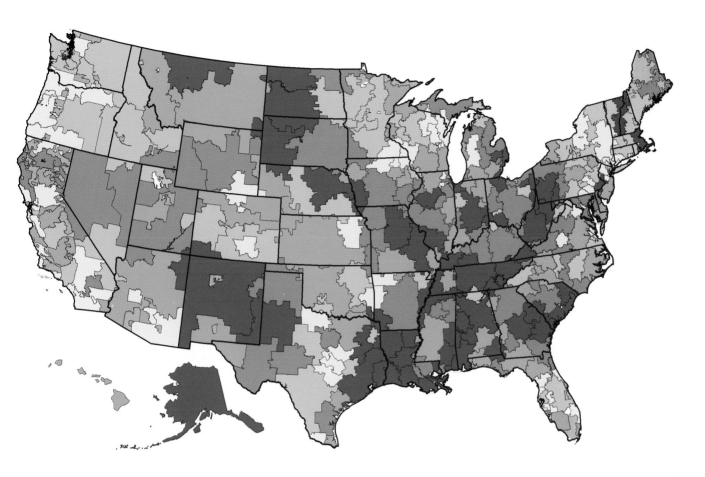

Map 2.4. Total Acute Care Hospital Expenditures

Hospital expenditures in 1993 were highest in the Midwest, South, and in metropolitan areas, with the exception of cities in California. Total inpatient and outpatient expenditures were generally lowest in California and the Pacific Northwest, and in some areas, like Minnesota, where managed care and other efforts to control costs have been effective.

Acute Care Hospital Expenditures per capita
by Hospital Referral Region (1993)

- ◼ $1,169 to 1,682 (61 HRRs)
- ◼ 1,062 to <1,169 (61)
- ◼ 978 to <1,062 (59)
- ◻ 895 to < 978 (62)
- ◻ 503 to < 895 (63)
- ◻ Not Populated

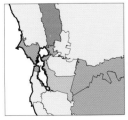

San Francisco

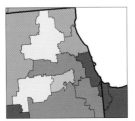

Chicago

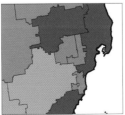

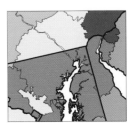

Detroit

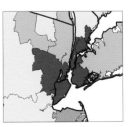

Washington-Baltimore

New York

PART THREE

Hospital Capacity, Utilization, and Outcomes

Hospital Capacity, Utilization, and Outcomes

The availability of hospital resources is linked to hospital expenditures. The greater the per capita supply of hospital resources, the greater will be their per capita use, and the greater the per capita expenditures. This relationship is both straightforward and easy to understand.

The relationship between hospital capacity and clinical decision making is more complex. In the absence of strong scientific evidence about the outcomes of interventions, physicians must act to solve patients' problems in the best way they know how. This frequently involves deciding whether or not the patient would be best served by being admitted to a hospital. The belief that hospitalization is efficacious is widely shared between patients and physicians. Most patients who are seriously ill willingly accept the recommendation that they be hospitalized; most physicians believe that such patients are better served with such care. These assumptions lead naturally to the use of available hospital resources, up to the point of their exhaustion. This is true in spite of the fact that the benefits of hospitalization for most conditions have not been tested by clinical studies.

The effect of capacity on utilization is evidenced by the fact that hospitals in areas with very high per capita supplies of hospital beds are as likely to have high occupancy rates as are hospitals in areas with low per capita supplies of hospital beds, even in areas that are demographically very similar. For example, the occupancy rate in Boston hospitals is about equal to the occupancy rate in New Haven hospitals, even though there are substantially more beds per capita in Boston than there are in New Haven, and in spite of the fact that the two cities are demographically much alike.

Hospital capacity is selective in its influence on clinical decision making. For the majority of common episodes of illness, patients obviously do not need hospitalization, and their treatments are not influenced by hospital capacity. Some patients have conditions, such as hip fracture, about which virtually all physicians agree on the diagnosis and the need for hospitalization. These patients find their way into the hospital, regardless of the number of beds per thousand residents. But only a minority of beds are occupied by patients who have conditions about which all physicians agree on the necessity for hospitalization. This is true even in areas with relatively few beds per thousand.

When the number of hospital beds per thousand residents increases, some of the incremental capacity is allocated to surgical cases; but most of the increased bed capacity is used to treat patients with a host of common acute and chronic medical illnesses, such as pneumonia, gastroenteritis, and chronic lung disease.

Hospital Capacity and Per Capita Expenditures for Hospital Care

In the early 1960s, Milton Roemer, a health services researcher interested in the use of hospitals, suggested that hospital beds, once built, will be used, no matter how many there are. The relationship between the capacity of the acute care hospital sector (measured in allocated beds per thousand residents of the local hospital referral region) and the costs of care provides an important illustration of what has become known as "Roemer's law." Figure 3.1 demonstrates the strong correlation (R^2=.57) between hospital beds per thousand residents and hospital expenditures per capita.

The number of hospital employees is another measure of hospital capacity. Figure 3.2 illustrates the relationship between the numbers of employees per thousand residents in hospital

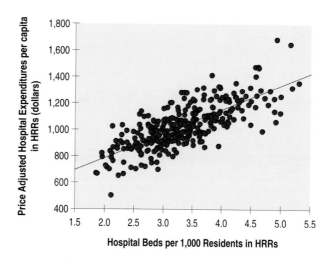

Figure 3.1. The Association Between Allocated Hospital Beds and Price Adjusted Hospital Expenditures (1993)

Greater hospital bed capacity per thousand residents of the hospital referral region is associated with higher expenditures per capita (R^2=.57). In the 33 regions with fewer than 2.5 beds per thousand residents, the average per capita expenditure was $831. In the 21 regions with more than 4.5 beds per thousand, the average per capita expenditure was $1,389, or 67% higher.

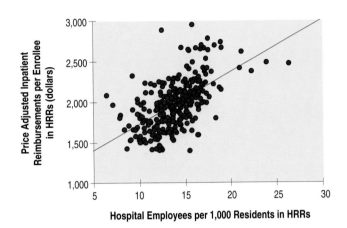

Figure 3.2. The Association Between Allocated Hospital Employees and Price Adjusted Medicare Reimbursements for Inpatient Hospital Services (1993)

Greater numbers of hospital employees per thousand residents of the hospital referral region are associated with higher Medicare reimbursements per enrollee ($R^2 = .32$). In the 20 regions with fewer than 10 full time equivalent hospital employees per thousand residents, the average per capita reimbursement was $1,773. In the 27 regions with more than 17 hospital employees per thousand, the average per capita reimbursement was $2,372, or 34% higher.

referral regions and the regions' price adjusted per enrollee reimbursements for acute care hospital services for the Medicare population. The numbers of full time equivalent hospital employees and Medicare reimbursements for acute hospital care are also correlated ($R^2 = .32$)

Hospital Capacity and Medicare Hospitalizations for Hip Fractures

Roemer's law does not apply equally to all conditions. Hospitalization rates for some injuries, such as hip fractures, and certain illnesses, such as heart attacks and major strokes, are not very sensitive to the hospital capacity; physicians everywhere appear to agree on the need to hospitalize all patients in whom these conditions are diagnosed.

It is easy to understand why the rate of hospitalization for hip fractures is closely related to the actual incidence of the condition. Hip fractures are life-threatening, and patients who break their hips almost always seek medical care. The condition is easily diagnosed with either physical examination or X-ray. Once hip fractures are diagnosed, virtually all patients are admitted to the hospital, even when beds are in short supply.

Hospital capacity has little influence on the rate of hospitalization of Medicare patients with hip fractures. Figure 3.3 shows the association between beds per thousand residents of hospital referral regions and the age, sex, and race adjusted rates of hospitalization. The correlation between them is weak (R^2=.07)

Conditions like hip fracture, about which virtually all physicians agree on the diagnosis and the need for hospitalization, are relatively rare. Patients with these conditions occupy a small proportion of the available beds – less than 20% – even in regions with low per capita hospital bed capacity.

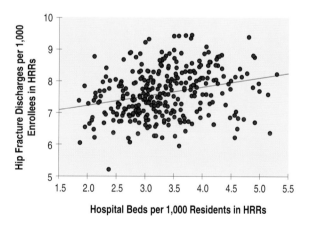

Figure 3.3. The Association Between Allocated Hospital Beds and Medicare Hospitalizations for Hip Fractures (1992-93)

There is little relationship between the hospital bed capacity and the discharge rate for hip fractures (R^2=.07). In hospital referral regions with more than 4.5 beds per thousand residents, the average discharge rate for hip fracture was 7.3; in regions with fewer than 2.5 beds per thousand, it was 7.2 per thousand Medicare enrollees.

Hospital Capacity and Medicare Hospitalizations for Surgical Care

About 30% of hospitalizations of Medicare enrollees involve surgery. In recent years, health policy makers have sought to promote the wider use of outpatient surgery as a means of controlling costs, yet Roemer's law still influences the rates of hospitalization for surgery. Figure 3.4 shows the association between beds per thousand residents and the age, sex, and race adjusted rates of Medicare surgical hospitalizations (R^2=.20). The relationship between capacity and the hospitalization rate is important, but not as strong as for medical conditions.

Previous studies have shown that the effect of capacity is largely on the admission rates for minor surgery – procedures that can be done on an outpatient basis. Major operations are not very sensitive to overall bed capacity. The rates of major surgery are influenced by other factors, including the per capita numbers of surgeons, the availability of diagnostic screening tests, and the practice styles of individual physicians.

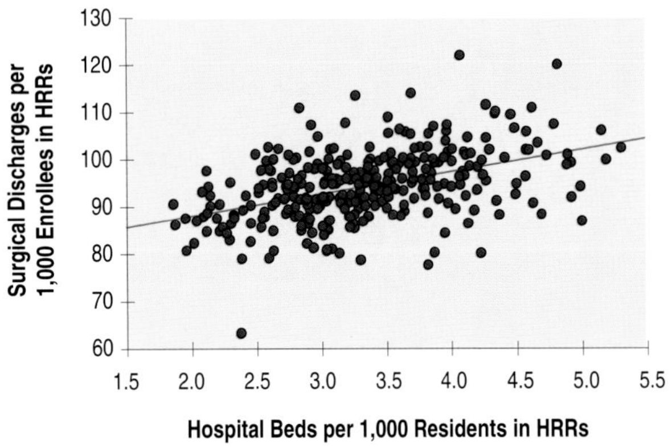

Figure 3.4. The Association Between Allocated Hospital Beds and Medicare Hospitalizations for Surgical Care (1992-93)

Hospital capacity is related to the Medicare discharge rate for surgical care. In hospital referral regions with fewer than 2.5 beds per thousand residents, the average discharge rate for surgical care among Medicare enrollees was 87.5 per thousand; in regions with more than 4.5 beds, it was 97.3.

Hospital Capacity and Medicare Hospitalizations for High Variation Medical Conditions

Most patients – more than 80% – who are admitted to the medical wards of the nation's hospitals are suffering with what have been described as "high variation medical conditions." These are conditions that show striking variation in the rates of admission among regions. They include such problems as pneumonia, chronic obstructive pulmonary disease, gastroenteritis, and congestive heart failure. Hospital capacity exercises its strongest influence on physicians' decisions about whether to hospitalize patients with such conditions.

Figure 3.5 demonstrates the strong relationship between hospital beds per thousand residents and the hospitalization rate for patients with high variation conditions (R^2=.57). In contrast to hip fracture patients, the rules used for decisions about whether or not to hospitalize patients with high variation medical conditions are not well standardized; there is no scientific basis for professional consensus. Physicians cannot consult medical textbooks to learn which patients with high variation medical conditions should be hospitalized and which could be safely treated outside the hospital. In areas with higher supplies of acute care hospital beds per thousand residents, people with high variation medical conditions are more likely to be admitted to the hospital than they would be if they had the same condition but were living in a region with lower per capita supplies of hospital beds. In the absence of consensus, availability drives utilization and costs.

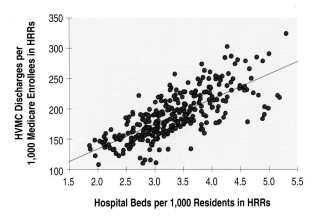

Figure 3.5. The Association Between Allocated Hospital Beds and Medicare Hospitalizations for High Variation Medical Conditions (1992-93)

There is a strong relationship between hospital capacity and its utilization for the treatment of patients with high variation medical conditions (R^2=.57). In hospital referral regions with fewer than 2.5 beds per thousand residents, the average discharge rate for patients with these conditions was 145.0 per thousand; in regions with more than 4.5 beds per thousand residents, the rate was 219.8.

Hospital Capacity and the Place Where Death Occurs

Hospital capacity influences the decisions physicians make about whether to hospitalize patients across a broad spectrum of disease. Studies in the 1980s comparing Boston (which had 4.5 beds per thousand residents) and New Haven (which had 2.9) illustrated that 22% of the residents of Boston enrolled in Medicare were admitted to hospitals; in New Haven, only 16% were. The threshold effect also works to increase the intensity of care of the very sick. In 1985, Medicare reimbursements for hospital care for patients who died in hospitals were 2.1 times greater per enrollee for Bostonians than for residents of New Haven. Forty percent of deaths of Bostonians occurred in hospitals, compared to 32% among Medicare enrollees living in New Haven.

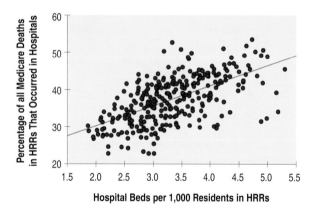

Hospital Beds per 1,000 Residents in HRRs

Researchers have found evidence that many elderly patients would prefer to die at home, rather than in a hospital, but hospital capacity has an important, and apparently overriding, bearing on the place where death occurs. Figure 3.6 illustrates the association between allocated hospital beds per thousand residents and the probability that deaths of Medicare enrollees will occur in a hospital. The R^2 is .36.

Figure 3.6. The Association Between Allocated Hospital Beds and the Percentage of Medicare Deaths That Occurred in Hospitals (1992-93)

Greater hospital capacity increases the likelihood that Medicare deaths will occur in the hospital (R^2 = .36). In the 33 regions with fewer than 2.5 beds per thousand residents, an average of 30.5% of all Medicare deaths occurred in a hospital. In the 21 regions with more than 4.5 beds per thousand residents, the rate was 1.52 times higher; an average of 46.6% of deaths occurred during a hospitalization.

Is More Better?

Residents of regions with higher hospital capacity experience greater use of hospital care, although the threshold effect of capacity on clinical decision making does not extend to all conditions, as illustrated in Figure 3.7. The strong link between the supply of resources, their utilization, and the amount expended on them, raises a crucial question: Do hospital referral regions with greater hospital capacity have better health outcomes?

While there are many dimensions of health outcomes, the easiest to measure and the most important for acute care hospital services is mortality. There is little evidence that populations living in communities or regions with higher resource investment in inpatient care have lower mortality. Epidemiologic studies relating level of use of hospital care to population-based mortality rates in New England failed to show lower mortality rates in high rate areas, even though hospital expenditures in some communities, such as Boston, were almost twice as high as in low use communities, such as New Haven. A recent national study conducted in conjunction with the research for the Atlas found a slight increase in mortality among hospital service areas with higher levels of investment in acute hospital care, even after controlling for age, sex, race, income, and a number of other factors related to illness and the need for care. Although correlations at the population level do not provide direct evidence of cause and effect, the association does not support the hypothesis that more hospital care results in lower population mortality rates.

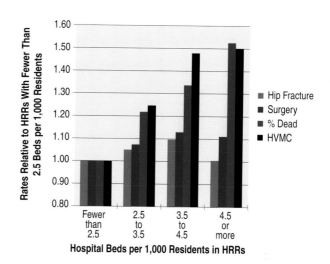

Figure 3.7. Summary of Effect of Hospital Capacity on Utilization (1992-93)

The threshold effect of capacity on clinical decision making does not extend to all conditions. The figure compares the hospitalization experience in regions with 2.5 beds per thousand or more to regions with fewer than 2.5 beds. There is no consistent relationship between hospital capacity and the discharge rate for hip fractures. The discharge rate for inpatient surgery increases as the number of beds increases. As hospital capacity increases, the greatest increases in utilization are seen in the discharge rates for high variation medical conditions and in the intensity of care for the very sick (measured here by the percentage of all Medicare deaths in the region that occurred in hospitals).

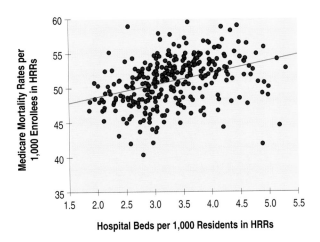

Figure 3.8. The Association Between Allocated Hospital Beds and Population Based Medicare Mortality

Mortality rates, after adjustment for age, sex, and race, tend to be higher in regions with greater numbers of allocated beds (R^2=.13). In the 33 regions with fewer than 2.5 beds per thousand residents, the population weighted and age, sex and race adjusted mortality rate was 49.4; in the 21 regions with more than 4.5 beds, the rate was 51.2.

Figure 3.8 examines the association between level of input of hospital resources and mortality. Among the 306 hospital referral regions, those with greater capacity, measured in numbers of hospital beds per capita, had higher age, sex, and race adjusted mortality (R^2=.13).

Hospital Capacity, Income Levels, and Medicare Hospitalizations for High Variation Medical Conditions

Health service researchers have long recognized that residents of lower income neighborhoods have higher rates of illness and of hospital utilization than those who live in more affluent areas. The association between income and utilization has been understood to be evidence that need drives utilization.

Research for the Atlas demonstrates an association between income level and utilization: Medicare residents living in low income neighborhoods (those with ZIP Code median incomes of less than $20,000) experience 41% more hospitalizations than those living in high income neighborhoods (those with ZIP Code median incomes of more than $40,000). Hospital capacity, however, has an effect on hospitalization rates that is independent of income. To examine this effect we compared rates of hospitalization for high variation medical conditions among the Medicare population according to the mean income in their neighborhoods and the capacity of the acute care hospital sector in their hospital referral regions .

We found that residents of high income neighborhoods in regions with high supplies of hospital beds actually had higher hospitalization rates than residents of low income neighborhoods in regions with low supplies of beds (177 hospitalizations for high variation conditions per thousand residents vs. 172 per thousand). Residents of low income neighborhoods in regions with high supplies of beds had hospitalization rates that were 56% higher than the rates for residents of low income neighborhoods in regions with low supplies of beds (Figure 3.9). Medicare enrollees living in moderate income ZIP Codes ($20,000-$40,000) within regions with high supplies of hospital beds had 45% higher admission rates than their counterparts in regions with low supplies of hospital beds. Similarly, residents of high income ZIP Codes in regions with high supplies of hospital beds had more than 30% more hospitalizations than residents of high income ZIP Codes in regions with low supplies of hospital beds.

Figure 3.9. The Association Between Hospital Capacity and Medicare Hospitalization Rates for High Variation Medical Conditions Among Populations, Stratified by Median Income in ZIP Code of Residence

Medicare patients were grouped according to the median income in the ZIP Code of their mailing addresses and according to the number of hospital beds per thousand residents in the hospital referral region to which their ZIP Code belonged. Hospitalization rates for high variation medical conditions were considerably higher in these regions than in regions with fewer beds. The largest difference was among those living in ZIP Codes with median incomes of less than $20,000, where the hospitalization rate for those living in regions with high supplies of beds was 56% greater than for those living in regions with fewer than 2.5 beds per thousand residents.

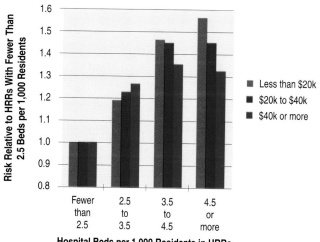

PART FOUR

The Medicare Program

The Medicare Program

In 1993, more than 34.0 million Americans over the age of 65 were enrolled in the Medicare program. Most – more than 32.4 million – received their care from "traditional" Medicare. That is, their care was obtained from providers who charged on a fee-for-service basis, either as independent practitioners or as members of health maintenance organizations that were not capitated. In 1993, $115.2 billion – over 95% of Medicare outlays for people over 65 – was reimbursed on a fee-for-service basis.

There were large differences in these reimbursements between hospital referral regions. Total program outlays per capita varied by a factor of more than two, even after adjusting for differences in prices among the regions. Price adjusted reimbursements for acute hospital care varied more than 2.1-fold, professional and laboratory services by more than 4.3, and home health care services by more than 25.0. The uneven distribution of reimbursements raises the question of whether areas with lower levels of acute care hospital services might have been achieving their inpatient savings by substituting outpatient care, hospice care, or home health care services. Research conducted in conjunction with the preparation of this Atlas shows very little evidence of substitution. The opposite is often the case. Regions with higher reimbursements for acute care hospital services tend also to have higher reimbursements for hospital-based outpatient care, as well as higher reimbursements for physician services and home health care services.

In 1993, approximately 1.6 million Medicare enrollees over the age of 65 were members of "new" Medicare – that is, "risk bearing" or capitated payment managed care plans. The Medicare program contributed about $7.7 billion in reimbursements for the care of these enrollees as contract payments to health maintenance organizations. There were large variations in the amount the federal government reimbursed for the care of those covered under the "new" Medicare, since payments were based on the fee-for-service reimbursement rate in the region where the beneficiary lived.

The proportion of Medicare beneficiaries who were enrolled in risk bearing managed care varied greatly among hospital referral regions. More than 59.8% of beneficiaries over the age of 65 lived in regions where less than 1% were members of risk bearing health maintenance organizations. In San Bernardino, California, and San Diego, California, more than 36% of Medicare participants were enrolled in health maintenance organizations. Regions with higher per capita reimbursements for traditional Medicare also tended to have larger proportions of Medicare enrollees in risk bearing health maintenance organizations.

Estimates for reimbursements are based on a 5% sample of the Medicare population as recorded in the Continuous Medicare History File. Fee-for-service reimbursements have been price adjusted to take into account differences in the cost of living among hospital referral regions.

Medicare Reimbursements for Traditional (Noncapitated) Medicare

In 1993, price adjusted Medicare payments for Americans over the age of 65 for services reimbursed on a fee-for-service basis (including non-risk bearing health maintenance organizations) amounted to $115.9 billion, an average of $3,929 per enrollee. Price adjusted per enrollee reimbursements varied remarkably among hospital referral regions. The region with the lowest rate of Medicare reimbursement was Lincoln, Nebraska, which had an average Medicare payment of $2,729 per enrollee in 1993; the hospital referral region with the highest rate was Miami, which was reimbursed $5,966 per enrollee – more than twice the rate in Lincoln.

Among the hospital referral regions with the highest per capita reimbursements for all services were, in addition to Miami, New Orleans ($5,391); Pittsburgh ($5,096); Nashville, Tennessee ($4,785); Baltimore ($4,664); Birmingham, Alabama ($4,643); Houston ($4,624); and Los Angeles ($4,615).

Among the large hospital referral regions with lower price adjusted Medicare reimbursements per capita were Honolulu ($2,917); Minneapolis ($2,984); Grand Rapids, Michigan ($3,066); Buffalo, New York ($3,100); Albany, New York ($3,173); Albuquerque, New Mexico ($3,178); San Jose, California ($3,211); and Arlington, Virginia ($3,218).

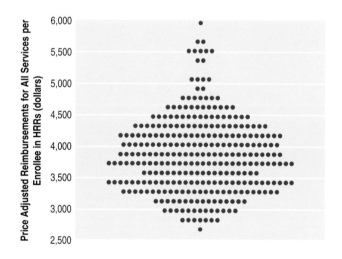

Figure 4.1. Price Adjusted Reimbursements for Traditional (Noncapitated) Medicare Among Hospital Referral Regions (1993)

Per enrollee reimbursements by the Medicare program for all services varied by a factor of more than 2, from about $2,700 to almost $6,000. Each point represents one of the 306 hospital referral regions in the United States.

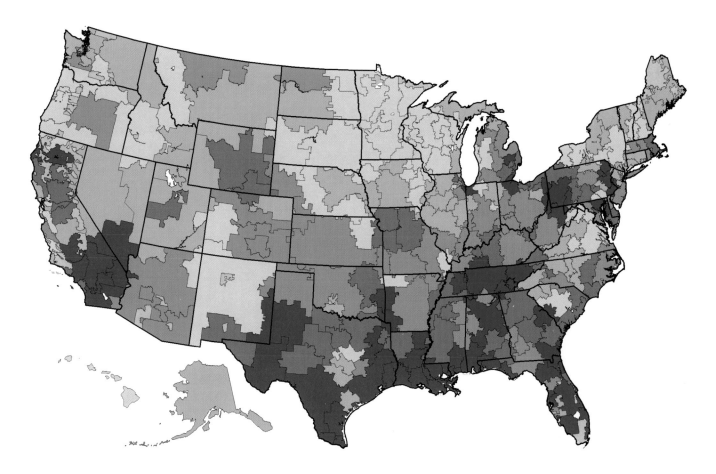

Map 4.1. Price Adjusted Reimbursements for Traditional (Noncapitated) Medicare

Total Medicare reimbursements for all services were generally higher in urban and densely populated areas and lower in more rural regions in 1993. Reimbursements were higher in the East, South, and West than in the Midwest and Northwest.

Total Medicare Reimbursements per Medicare Enrollee
by Hospital Referral Region (1993)

- $4,340 to 5,966 (61 HRRs)
- 4,020 to <4,340 (61)
- 3,702 to <4,020 (61)
- 3,336 to <3,702 (61)
- 2,729 to <3,336 (62)
- Not Populated

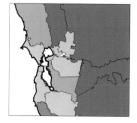

San Francisco

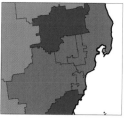

Chicago

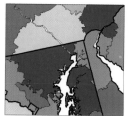

Detroit

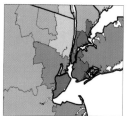

Washington-Baltimore

New York

Medicare Reimbursements for Professional and Laboratory Services

Professional services reimbursements include payments to surgeons and medical doctors for activities such as office consultations, vaccinations, and open heart surgery. Among the more common laboratory services are biopsy evaluations and blood tests. In 1993, price adjusted reimbursements for fee-for-service professional and laboratory services for Americans over age 65 totaled $31.2 billion, an average of $1,057 per enrollee. This represented 26.9% of total price adjusted Medicare outlays for traditional Medicare.

With price adjusted reimbursements for professional and laboratory services totaling $2,380 per enrollee, Miami had the highest rate in the United States. Los Angeles, with per capita reimbursements of $1,575, was substantially lower than Miami, but four times higher than the lowest rate region. Other regions with high per enrollee reimbursements included Fort Lauderdale, Florida ($1,559); Orange County, California ($1,449); Manhattan ($1,325); Detroit ($1,302); Philadelphia ($1,309); San Diego ($1,361); Tampa, Florida ($1,311); New Orleans ($1,310); and Baltimore ($1,200).

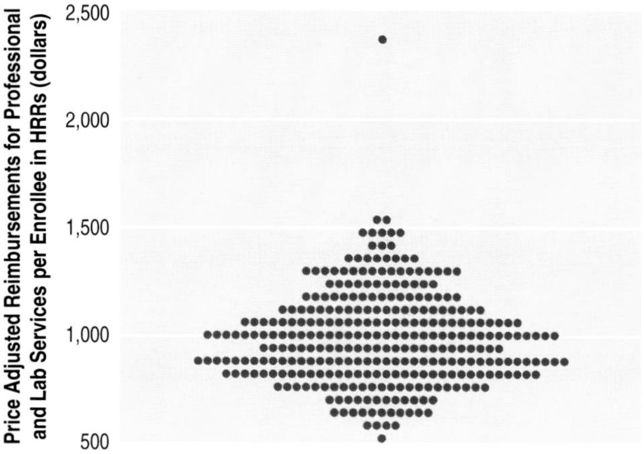

Among the regions with relatively low per capita reimbursements for professional and laboratory services were Minneapolis ($585); Madison, Wisconsin ($671); Rochester, Minnesota ($671); Portland, Oregon ($729); Sioux Falls, South Dakota ($738); Salt Lake City ($748); Rochester, New York ($780); and Albuquerque, New Mexico ($809).

Figure 4.2. Price Adjusted Part B Medicare Reimbursements for Professional and Laboratory Services Among Hospital Referral Regions (1993)

Reimbursements for professional and laboratory services varied by a factor of more than 4, from $546 per Medicare enrollee to $2,380. Each point represents one of the 306 hospital referral regions in the United States.

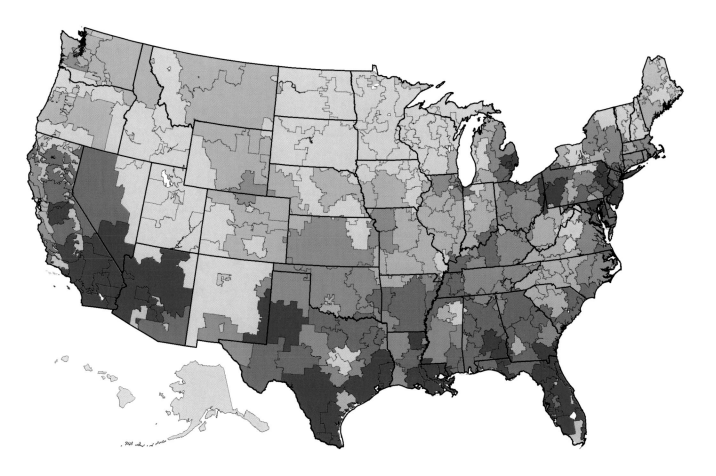

Map 4.2. Price Adjusted Medicare Reimbursements for Professional and Laboratory Services

Reimbursements for fee-for-service professional and laboratory services were highest in the South and on the West Coast; Florida and the Mid-Atlantic region also had high reimbursements. Some areas, including Texas, had wide variations among hospital referral regions within the state.

Reimbursements for Professional and Laboratory Services per Medicare Enrollee
by Hospital Referral Region (1993)

- $1,170 to 2,380 (60 HRRs)
- 1,034 to <1,170 (62)
- 920 to <1,034 (61)
- 827 to < 920 (61)
- 546 to < 827 (62)
- Not Populated

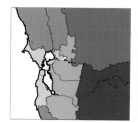

San Francisco

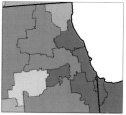

Chicago

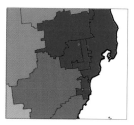

Detroit

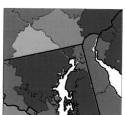

Washington-Baltimore

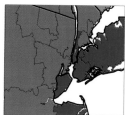

New York

Medicare Reimbursements for Inpatient Hospital Services

In 1993, price adjusted Medicare reimbursements to hospitals for acute, short stay care for Americans over age 65 whose care was paid for on a fee-for-service basis was $59.5 billion, or $2,018 per enrollee. These payments represented 51.4% of the Medicare program's total outlays for traditional Medicare. Price adjusted reimbursements to hospitals per Medicare enrollee were more than twice as high in the highest rate hospital referral region, Slidell, Louisiana ($2,956), than in the lowest rate region, Albuquerque, New Mexico ($1,407).

Among the large hospital referral regions with the highest rates of per enrollee reimbursements for acute hospital care were Pittsburgh ($2,786); Baltimore ($2,656); the Bronx, New York ($2,476); Toledo, Ohio ($2,423); and Chicago ($2,420). Other areas where per enrollee reimbursements for hospital care were high included Manhattan ($2,382); Philadelphia ($2,379); Houston ($2,347); and Miami ($2,297).

Other large metropolitan hospital referral regions had relatively low per enrollee payments for acute hospital care; they included Arlington, Virginia ($1,543); Honolulu ($1,558); Buffalo, New York ($1,601); San Francisco ($1,627); and Hartford, Connecticut ($1,647).

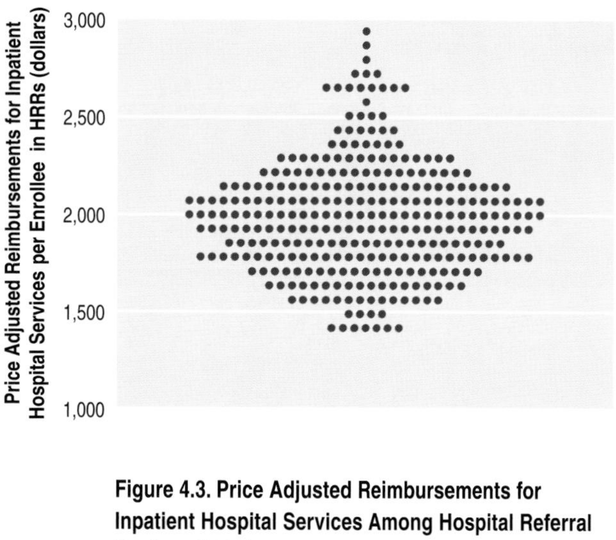

Figure 4.3. Price Adjusted Reimbursements for Inpatient Hospital Services Among Hospital Referral Regions (1993)

Per enrollee Medicare reimbursements for acute care hospital services varied by a factor of more than 2, from about $1,400 to almost $3,000. Each point represents one of the 306 hospital referral regions in the United States.

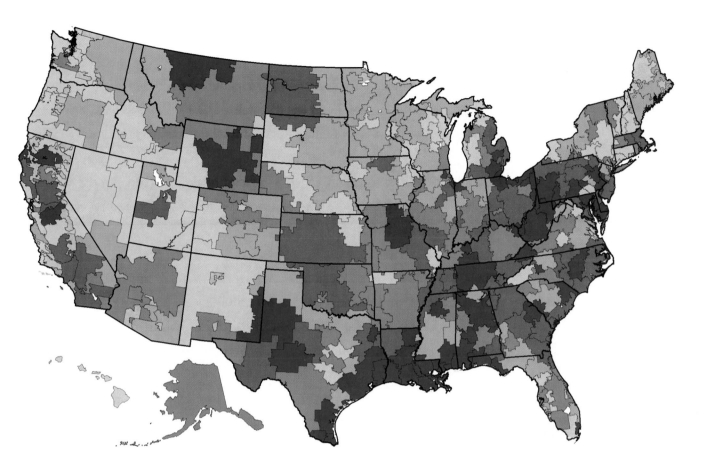

Map 4.3. Price Adjusted Medicare Reimbursements for Inpatient Hospital Services

Medicare reimbursements for inpatient hospital services were generally lower in the West than in the East, and generally higher in the South than elsewhere. Some high states, including Texas and Florida, had hospital referral regions with inpatient reimbursement rates in each of the five quintiles.

Reimbursements for Inpatient Hospital Services per Medicare Enrollee
by Hospital Referral Region (1993)

- $2,200 to 2,956 (63 HRRs)
- 2,036 to <2,200 (61)
- 1,893 to <2,036 (59)
- 1,732 to <1,893 (60)
- 1,407 to <1,732 (63)
- Not Populated

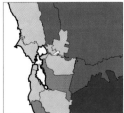

San Francisco

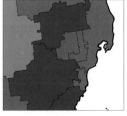

Chicago

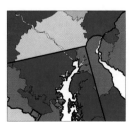

Detroit

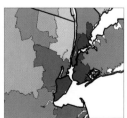

Washington-Baltimore

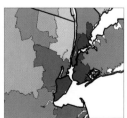

New York

Medicare Reimbursements for Outpatient Facilities

In 1993, price adjusted Medicare reimbursements for the use of fee-for-service outpatient facilities by enrollees over age 65 totaled $10.1 billion, or $342 per enrollee. These reimbursements represented 8.7% of total outlays for traditional Medicare.

Price adjusted reimbursements varied by a factor of almost 3 between the lowest rate hospital referral region, Sun City, Arizona ($190), and the highest rate region, Slidell, Louisiana ($552).

Among the hospital referral regions with the highest rates of price adjusted Medicare reimbursements for outpatient services per enrollee were Baltimore ($473); Omaha, Nebraska ($458); Toledo, Ohio ($442); Wichita, Kansas ($439); Ann Arbor, Michigan ($432); and Albuquerque, New Mexico ($430).

Among the hospital referral regions with relatively low per enrollee rates of reimbursement for outpatient services in 1993 were New Brunswick, New Jersey ($215); White Plains, New York ($226); East Long Island, New York ($226); Las Vegas ($232); Melrose Park, Illinois ($254); Honolulu ($255); and Columbia, South Carolina ($261).

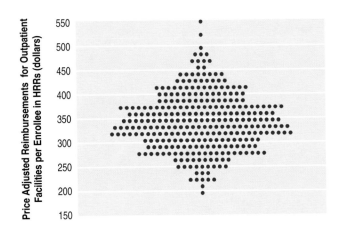

Figure 4.4. Price Adjusted Medicare Reimbursements for Outpatient Services Among Hospital Referral Regions (1993)

Price adjusted Medicare reimbursements for outpatient services varied by a factor of almost 3, from $190 per enrollee to $552. Each point represents one of the 306 hospital referral regions in the United States.

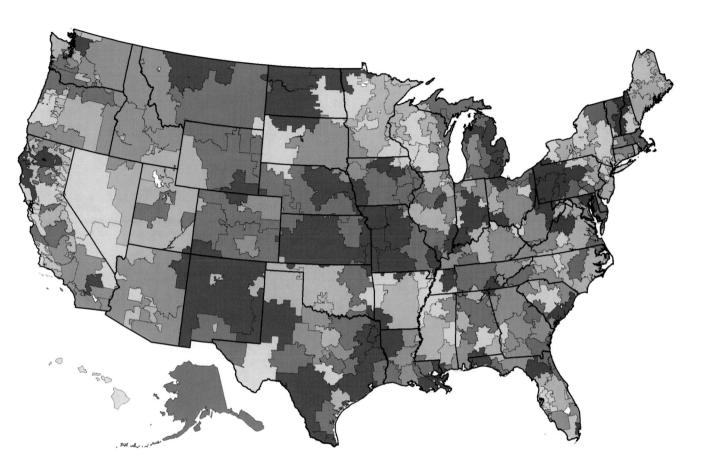

Map 4.4. Price Adjusted Medicare Reimbursements for Outpatient Services

Outpatient facilities were most heavily used in urban areas, particularly in New England and the West Coast, and in parts of the Midwest and Southwest. In New Mexico, Texas, and parts of the Midwest, regions with high rates of use of outpatient facilities were contiguous with regions with low rates; in many areas, rates of use of inpatient and outpatient facilities were both high.

Reimbursements for Outpatient Facilities per Medicare Enrollee
by Hospital Referral Region (1993)

- $393 to 552 (61 HRRs)
- 356 to <393 (61)
- 326 to <356 (61)
- 291 to <326 (61)
- 190 to <291 (62)
- Not Populated

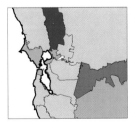

San Francisco

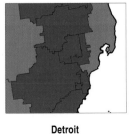

Chicago

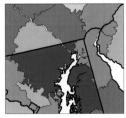

Detroit

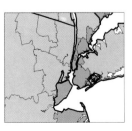

Washington-Baltimore

New York

Medicare Reimbursements for Home Health Care Services

In 1993, price adjusted Medicare reimbursements for home health care services for enrollees over age 65 paid for on a fee-for-service basis totaled $9.24 billion, or $313 per enrollee. These reimbursements represented 8.0% of traditional Medicare program outlays.

Variations in the levels of Medicare reimbursements for home health care were extreme. The highest price adjusted reimbursement rate per Medicare enrollee, in Chattanooga, Tennessee ($1,292), was 25 times higher than that in Rochester, Minnesota, which had the lowest rate ($51).

The per capita reimbursement for Medicare enrollees in the Chattanooga hospital referral region was 25% higher than in the next highest region, Baton Rouge, Louisiana ($1,032). Other parts of Tennessee, including Knoxville ($975), Nashville ($966), Jackson ($856), Johnson City ($629), and Memphis ($574), were also very high.

Other parts of the South also had high per enrollee home health reimbursements, including Jackson, Mississippi ($710); New Orleans ($700); Miami ($612); Birmingham, Alabama ($550); and Orlando, Florida ($543).

Among the hospital referral regions with the lowest per capita rates of reimbursement were Minneapolis ($102); Wichita, Kansas ($124); White Plains, New York ($130); Hackensack, New Jersey ($136); Honolulu ($139); Morristown, New Jersey ($140); and Richmond, Virginia ($162).

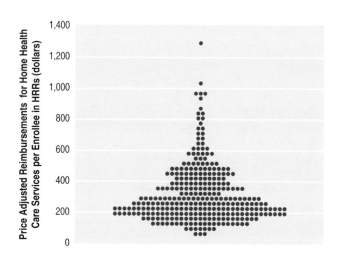

Figure 4.5. Price Adjusted Medicare Reimbursements for Home Health Care Services Among Hospital Referral Regions (1993)

Price adjusted Medicare reimbursements for home health care services varied by a factor of 25, from $51 per enrollee to almost $1300. Each point represents one of the 306 hospital referral regions in the United States.

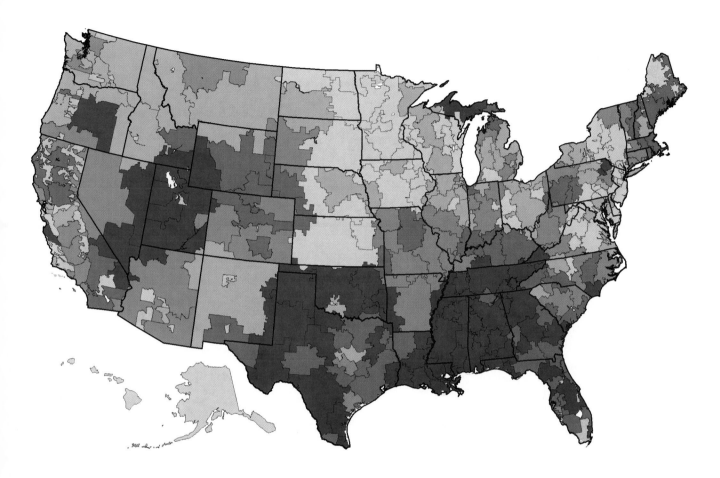

Map 4.5. Price Adjusted Medicare Reimbursements for Home Health Care Services

Home health care services were more heavily used in the South and West than elsewhere in the country; in contrast to most other health care services, home health care was less heavily utilized in urban areas than in rural regions. The Upper Midwest and Northwest had notably low rates of use of home health care services.

Reimbursements for Home Health Care Services per Medicare Enrollee
by Hospital Referral Region (1993)

- $451 to 1,292 (63 HRRs)
- 305 to <451 (59)
- 235 to <305 (60)
- 189 to <235 (62)
- 51 to <189 (62)
- Not Populated

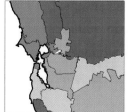
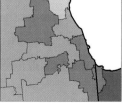
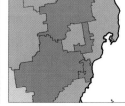
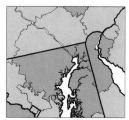
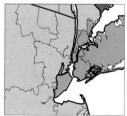

San Francisco   Chicago   Detroit   Washington-Baltimore   New York

Are There Tradeoffs Between Sectors of Care?

It has often been proposed that overall expenditures for health care can be reduced by substituting less costly care, such as hospital outpatient services and home health care, for more costly hospital inpatient care. It has also been suggested that reimbursements for physicians' services might be lower in regions with greater use of home health care services. Others theorize that regions with relatively scarce per capita investment in physician services have higher costs for hospital care. The documented patterns of variation in reimbursements for Medicare services provide no evidence that such substitutions are occurring.

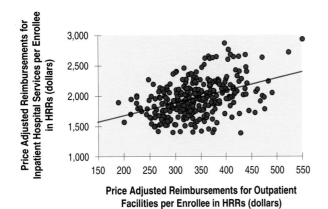

Price Adjusted Reimbursements for Outpatient Facilities per Enrollee in HRRs (dollars)

Figure 4.6. The Association Between Price Adjusted Medicare Reimbursements for Outpatient and Inpatient Hospital Services (1993)

Regions with higher reimbursements for outpatient care tended to have higher inpatient reimbursements ($R^2 = .17$).

Greater levels of expenditures for outpatient services were not associated with lower levels of expenditure for inpatient services. Indeed, the opposite is the case: regions with higher levels of reimbursement for outpatient care tended to have higher reimbursements for acute hospital care (Figure 4.6).

A number of regions that were in the top 20% of spending for outpatient services were also in the top quintile for spending on inpatient care; examples include Slidell, Louisiana, which ranks first in inpatient as well as outpatient reimbursements among the 306 hospital referral regions. Johnstown, Pennsylvania, ranks fourth in inpatient and second in outpatient reimbursements. Among larger hospital referral regions that rank in the top quintile for both inpatient and outpatient reimbursements are Ann Arbor, Michigan; Baltimore; and Houston.

Similarly, several regions in the lowest 20% of reimbursements for inpatient care were also in the lowest 20% for outpatient care. These included Buffalo, New York; Albany, New York; Hackensack, New Jersey; and Honolulu. Albuquerque, New Mexico, was the exception. It ranked lowest among the 306 regions in inpatient cost and was among the top 10% in outpatient reimbursements.

There was also no evidence of tradeoffs between other alternatives to acute hospital care and inpatient care. No association was found between the level of reimbursement for acute hospital care and for home health agency care (R^2=.03), hospice care (R^2=.00), or long stay care (R^2=.01)

Greater reimbursements for home health agency services were not associated with lower physician reimbursements. Indeed, there was a weak association in the opposite direction (R^2=.11), indicating that there may in fact be some relationship between higher rates of use of physicians' services and higher rates of use of home health care services.

Regions with higher reimbursements for physicians' services tended also to have higher reimbursements for acute hospital care. Figure 4.7 illustrates the correlation between price adjusted Medicare reimbursements for inpatient hospital services and price adjusted reimbursements for professional and laboratory services; the association has an R^2 of .23.

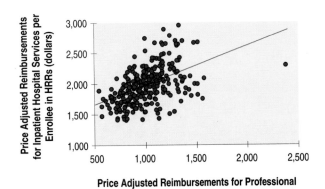

Figure 4.7. The Association Between Price Adjusted Medicare Reimbursements for Professional and Laboratory Services and for Inpatient Hospital Services (1993)

Communities with greater per enrollee outlays for short term hospitals tend also to have higher reimbursements for professional and laboratory services (R^2 =.23).

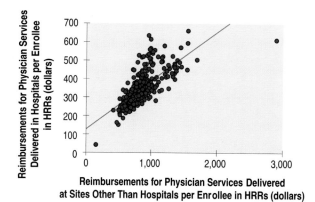

Figure 4.8. The Association Between Price Adjusted Medicare Part B Reimbursements for Professional and Laboratory Services Provided Outside and Inside the Hospital (1993)

Regions with higher Part B physician reimbursements for outpatient care tend to have higher Part B physician inpatient reimbursements (R^2 = .52).

Regions with higher Medicare Part B reimbursements for inpatient professional and laboratory services tended also to have higher reimbursements for these services provided outside the hospital (Figure 4.8). Part B reimbursements per Medicare enrollee for services provided in the hospital varied more than fourfold among the 306 regions; reimbursements for care provided at other sites also varied more than fourfold. The correlation between Medicare Part B reimbursements for inpatient care and care provided elsewhere has an R^2 of .52.

Medicare Enrollment in Capitated Managed Care Plans

Since the early 1970s, Medicare beneficiaries have been offered the option of joining risk bearing, or capitated, health maintenance organizations. Under the capitation plan, the federal government pays health maintenance organizations a fixed annual amount per enrollee. In exchange, the health maintenance organization must provide all required services. If the total costs of care exceed the amount the government pays, then the health maintenance organization must absorb the loss; if they are less, then the health maintenance organization may retain the difference.

In 1993, about 1.6 million, or 5.2%, of all Medicare enrollees were covered by risk bearing health maintenance organizations, but enrollment was geographically very uneven across the United States. More than 50% of those with health maintenance organization coverage lived in just eight hospital referral regions. Six were on the West Coast: Los Angeles; San Diego; San Bernardino, California; Orange County, California; Seattle; and Portland, Oregon. Two, Fort Lauderdale and Miami, were in Florida.

San Bernardino, California, where 50% of Medicare enrollees were in risk bearing health maintenance organizations, had the highest penetration, followed by San Diego (36%), Orange County (35%), and Portland (32%).

More than 60% of the Medicare population lived in hospital referral regions where less than 1% of beneficiaries were in risk bearing health maintenance organizations.

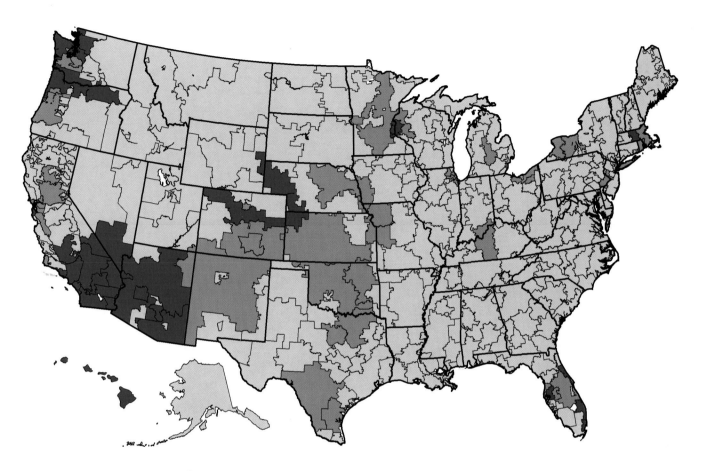

Map 4.6. Medicare Enrollment in Capitated Managed Care Plans

In some hospital referral regions, 15% or more of the resident Medicare population were members of risk bearing health maintenance organizations in 1993 (dark green). More than 71% of Medicare beneficiaries who were members of risk bearing health maintenance organizations lived in these regions. In other hospital referral regions, very few – less than 1% – of the Medicare population were enrolled in risk bearing health maintenance organizations (pale green).

Percentage of Medicare Population Enrolled in Risk Bearing HMOs
by Hospital Referral Region (1993)

- 15 or More   (24 HRRs)
- 1 to 15   (50)
- Less than 1   (232)
- Not Populated

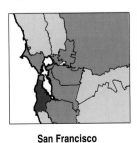

San Francisco

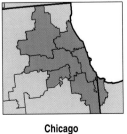

Chicago

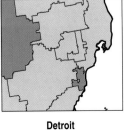

Detroit

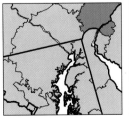

Washington-Baltimore

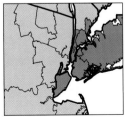

New York

The Federal Contribution for Medicare Enrollment in Risk Bearing Health Maintenance Organizations

The federal payment for managed care coverage of Medicare enrollees is based on the amount reimbursed for fee-for-service care where the enrollee lives. As a result, per enrollee reimbursements are significantly higher for managed care coverage in regions where reimbursements have historically been high. The difference can be substantial; for example, in 1993, the age, sex and race adjusted per enrollee Medicare reimbursement for residents of Minneapolis served by fee-for-service care was $2,794, while the per enrollee reimbursement for those living in Miami was $6,429, more than twice as much.

The amount of the federal reimbursement for managed care coverage has an obvious effect on the benefits that a managed care plan is able to offer Medicare enrollees. Health maintenance organizations in Miami or Los Angeles, where the reimbursement is well above the national average, can afford to offer such benefits as drugs, eyeglasses, and long term care. Health maintenance organizations in Minneapolis or in Rochester, Minnesota, where reimbursements are well below the national average, may not have the resources to provide such benefits. Enrollees living in historically efficient markets lose, while those in inefficient markets gain. Moreover, because the contributions that Americans make to the Medicare program have never been adjusted for regional costs, those in more efficient, low cost markets such as Minneapolis are subsidizing the care of those living in high cost regions like Miami.

What can be done to achieve geographic equity? The federal reimbursement can be adjusted to equalize the per enrollee federal payment in each region. Many parts of the country would benefit from such a policy. In 1993, 31 states had Medicare spending rates below the national average; in 10 states the rate was more than 25% below average.

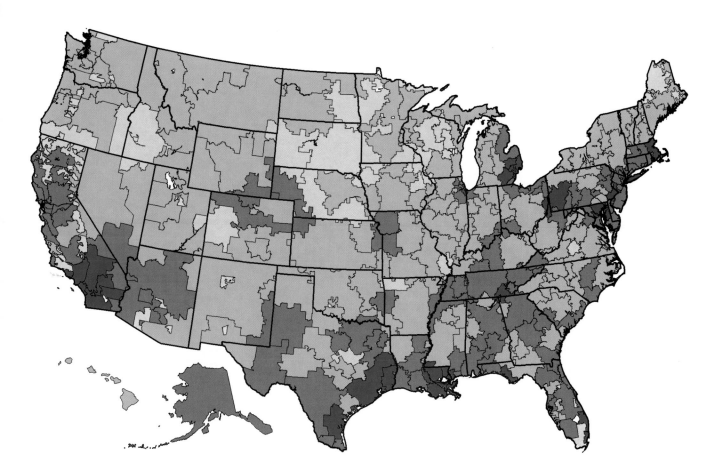

Map 4.7. Variations in Medicare Reimbursements

Hospital referral regions that have historically received reimbursements of less than 75% of the national average (lightest green) would benefit most from a policy to equalize differences in per enrollee reimbursements in establishing the value of the Medicare voucher. Those spending 125% or more of the national average would lose the most. Equalization would eliminate subsidies that now flow from residents of low cost regions to those in high cost regions.

Total Medicare Reimbursements as Percentage of U.S. Average
by Hospital Referral Region (1993)

- 125 to 176% (35 HRRs)
- 100 to <125% (104)
- 75 to <100% (146)
- 60 to < 75% (21)
- Not Populated

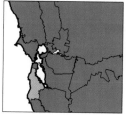

San Francisco

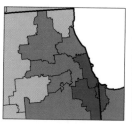

Chicago

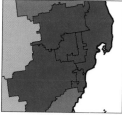

Detroit

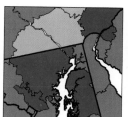

Washington-Baltimore

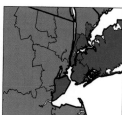

New York

PART FIVE

The Physician Workforce

This section provides measures of the allocation of physician resources to the populations living in the nation's 306 hospital referral regions. The data come from the American Medical Association, the American Osteopathic Association, and the Medicare program and are for 1993. A clinically active physician is defined as one who reported that he or she spends at least 20 hours a week in patient care. The population count is from the 1990 census.

The estimates for the physician workforce per 100,000 population take into account patient migration across the boundaries of the regions, using a method similar to that used for hospital beds (Part Two), except that surgical specialists are allocated on the basis of surgical admissions, and medical specialists and primary care physicians on the basis of medical admissions.

The estimates have been adjusted for differences in age and sex of the population. Part Nine explains how these adjustments were done.

The Physician Workforce Active in Patient Care

In the 1960s and early 1970s, American health care policy leaders believed that the physician workforce in the United States was inadequate, particularly in underserved areas. A concerted effort was undertaken to increase the number of medical schools and the size of their graduating classes. Residency programs were expanded and graduates of foreign medical schools were offered more opportunities to enter practice in the United States. These initiatives were extremely successful in increasing the size of the physician workforce. In 1970, there were 235,241 active physicians in the United States. By 1993, the number of active physicians had doubled, to 469,603. The supply of physicians increased by 67%, from 113.1 per hundred thousand persons in the United States to 189.0. (These figures measure physicians in active clinical practice and do not include physicians in residency training programs, who are counted separately.)

Despite this increase in the number of active physicians, there is still a great deal of geographic variation in the distribution of the workforce. Among the hospital referral regions with the highest total age and sex adjusted numbers of active physicians per hundred thousand residents in 1993 were San Francisco (317.2); White Plains, New York (303.8); Washington, D.C. (291.1); Hackensack, New Jersey (266.0); Manhattan (265.7); Philadelphia (259.4); and Boston (256.0). Regions that were below the United States average included Wichita, Kansas (142.9); Charlotte, North Carolina (149.0); Memphis, Tennessee (150.4); Columbus, Ohio (153.6); Fort Worth, Texas (154.4); Birmingham, Alabama (154.9); and Lexington, Kentucky (155.5).

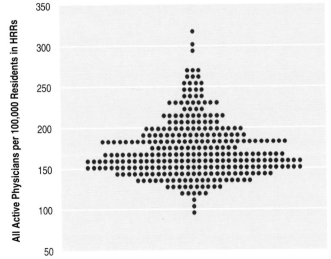

Figure 5.1. Physicians Allocated to Hospital Referral Regions (1993)

The number of physicians in active practice per hundred thousand residents, after adjusting for differences in age and sex of the local population, ranged from fewer than 100 to more than 300. Each point represents one of the 306 hospital referral regions in the United States.

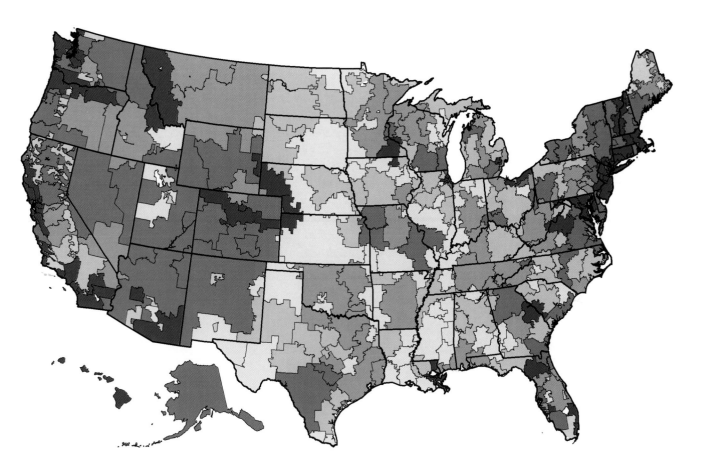

Map 5.1. The Physician Workforce Active in Patient Care

In 1993, there were higher numbers of physicians per hundred thousand residents on the East and West Coasts, parts of the Mountain States, and in the Pacific Northwest. Some regions with very high supplies of physicians were contiguous with areas that had much lower supplies, as in Kansas, Nebraska, and Louisiana.

Physicians per 100,000 Residents
by Hospital Referral Region (1993)

- 200.3 to 317.2 (61 HRRs)
- 178.4 to <200.3 (61)
- 159.2 to <178.4 (61)
- 145.7 to <159.2 (61)
- 92.5 to <145.7 (62)
- Not Populated

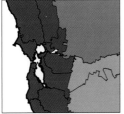

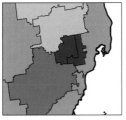

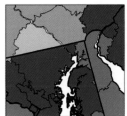

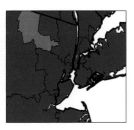

San Francisco   **Chicago**   **Detroit**   **Washington-Baltimore**   **New York**

Physicians in Primary Care

The number of active physicians in primary care practice increased by 62% between 1970 and 1993, from 101,251 to 164,146. The physician-to-population ratio increased by 36%, from 48.7 to 66.0 primary care physicians per hundred thousand residents of the United States. Among hospital referral regions, the supply of physicians clinically active in primary care in 1993 varied from 35.4 per hundred thousand residents in Harlingen, Texas, to 116.6 in San Francisco.

Among the hospital referral regions with the highest number of primary care physicians per hundred thousand residents were White Plains, New York (93.7); East Long Island, New York (92.3); Hackensack, New Jersey (90.0); Washington, D.C. (89.6); Philadelphia (89.3); Manhattan (88.6); Seattle (88.3); Alameda County, California (86.8); and Chicago (85.9).

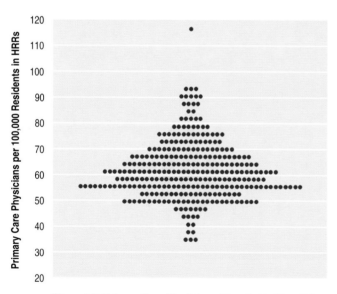

Figure 5.2. Primary Care Physicians Allocated to Hospital Referral Regions (1993)

The number of primary care physicians in active practice per hundred thousand residents, after adjusting for differences in age and sex of the local population, ranged from fewer than 36 to more than 116. Each point represents one of the 306 hospital referral regions in the United States.

Among the regions where the supply of primary care physicians per hundred thousand residents was lowest were El Paso, Texas (43.4); Winston-Salem, North Carolina (49.4); Charlotte, North Carolina (50.3); Memphis, Tennessee (50.7); Fort Worth, Texas (53.9); Binghamton, New York (54.9); San Bernardino, California (55.0); Dallas (56.2); and Houston (56.2).

There were only 24 hospital referral regions in the United States in 1993 that had fewer primary care physicians per hundred thousand population than the 1970 national average.

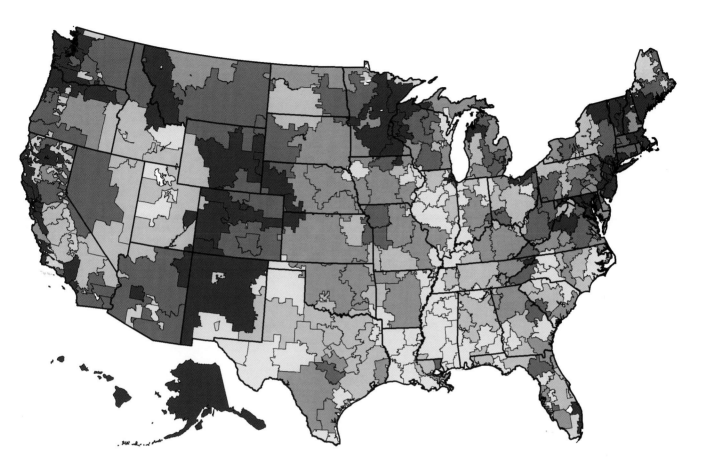

Map 5.2. Physicians in Primary Care

In 1993, the numbers of primary care physicians per hundred thousand residents were greatest in the Northeast, on the West Coast, and in the West.

**Primary Care Physicians
per 100,000 Residents**
by Hospital Referral Region (1993)

- 70.6 to 116.6 (62 HRRs)
- 62.9 to <70.6 (62)
- 57.4 to <62.9 (58)
- 53.7 to <57.4 (58)
- 35.4 to <53.7 (66)
- Not Populated

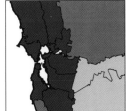

San Francisco

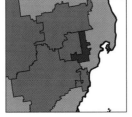

Chicago

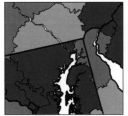

Detroit

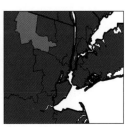

Washington-Baltimore

New York

Specialist Physicians

As the nation's medical schools produced more graduates, and foreign medical graduates were attracted to the United States in increasing numbers, the Medicare program provided the financing that made it possible for virtually all young physicians to become qualified in the specialty of their choice. The result was an increase in the number and proportion of physicians who practice specialty medicine and surgery. In 1970 there were 130,784 clinically active physicians who were identified as specialists; by 1993 the number had increased by a factor of 2.3, to 302,511. The population ratio also doubled, from 62.9 to 121.7 specialists per hundred thousand residents of the United States.

Among the areas with the highest numbers of specialists per hundred thousand residents were White Plains, New York (208.6); Washington, D.C. (198.9); San Francisco (196.8); Manhattan (175.6); Hackensack, New Jersey (174.3); and East Long Island, New York (171.0). The per capita numbers of specialists serving the populations of White Plains and Washington were about 60% higher than the national average.

Although some areas were far below the 1993 national average supply of specialists, only one hospital referral region in the country – McAllen, Texas (56.3) – had fewer specialists per capita in 1993 than the national average in 1970. Wichita, Kansas (80.2); Springfield, Illinois (85.7); Des Moines, Iowa (87.8); Cedar Rapids, Iowa (87.8); and Dayton, Ohio (89.8) were among the hospital referral regions with fewer than 100 specialists per hundred thousand population.

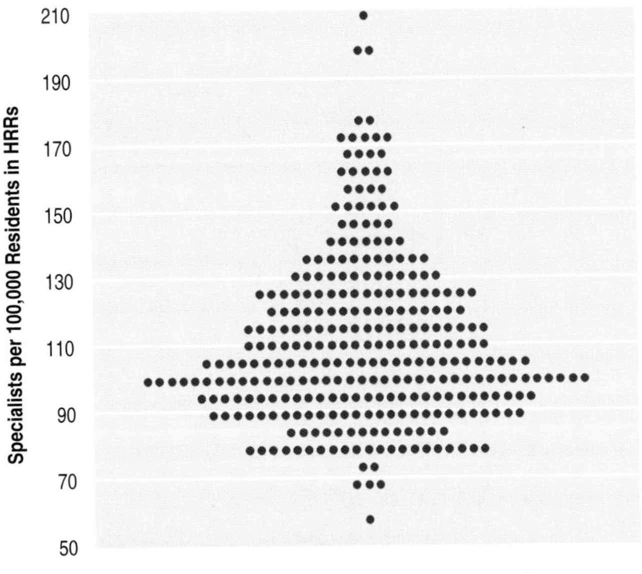

Figure 5.3. Specialists Allocated to Hospital Referral Regions (1993)

The number of specialist physicians in active practice per hundred thousand residents, after adjusting for differences in age and sex of the local population, ranged from about 56 to more than 200. Each point represents one of the 306 hospital referral regions in the United States.

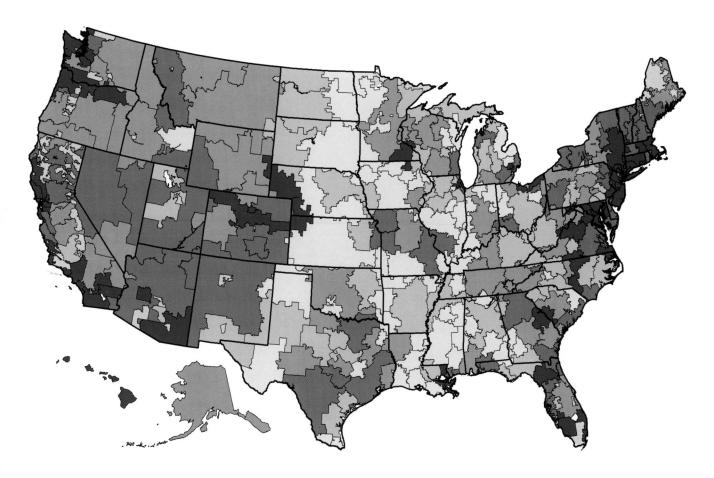

Map 5.3. Specialist Physicians

In 1993, the numbers of specialists per hundred thousand residents were highest on the East and West Coasts and lowest in the South and parts of the Midwest. Areas with higher than average supplies of specialists also included the Mountain States and parts of Texas.

Specialist Physicians per 100,000 Residents
by Hospital Referral Region (1993)

■ 128.7 to 208.6 (63 HRRs)
■ 111.9 to <128.7 (59)
■ 100.2 to <111.9 (60)
■ 90.8 to <100.2 (60)
□ 56.3 to < 90.8 (64)
□ Not Populated

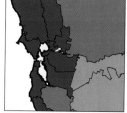

San Francisco

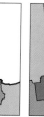

Chicago

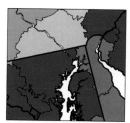

Detroit

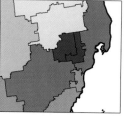

Washington-Baltimore

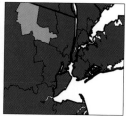

New York

The 50/50 Rule

Some health workforce analysts believe that the national goal should be a physician workforce that is equally balanced between specialists and primary care physicians. One argument for the "50/50 rule" is that it reflects the balance between specialists and primary physicians in other industrialized nations, such as Canada, and is similar to the balance in some staff-model health maintenance organizations.

How far is the nation from achieving the goal of a 50/50 distribution of specialists and generalists? In 1970, 44% of practicing physicians were in primary care. Although the total number of primary care physicians in active practice increased by 62% between 1970 and 1993, the total number of specialists increased even more. By 1993, only 35% of clinically active physicians in the United States were in primary care, and the proportion of active physicians who were in primary care ranged from 27.5% in New Orleans to 46.6% in Grand Forks, North Dakota.

Among regions with high percentages of generalists were Wichita, Kansas (43.6%): Minneapolis (41.3%); Tulsa, Oklahoma (39.4%); Lexington, Kentucky (39.2%); Spokane, Washington (39.2%); and Dayton, Ohio (38.8). In other hospital referral regions, less than one-third of the physician workforce was in generalist practice in 1993; among them were New Orleans (27.5%); White Plains, New York (31.0%); Washington, D.C. (31.1%); Salt Lake City (31.3%); Durham, North Carolina (31.5%); and San Antonio (31.6%).

The distribution of physicians between primary care and specialty care tells only part of the story. Some hospital referral regions had per capita supplies of both specialists and generalists in 1993 that were relatively low, and some areas had relatively high supplies of both. Simply raising the number or proportion of physicians in primary care in local markets does not address the question of whether the overall supply of primary care physicians in the community is high, low, or in between.

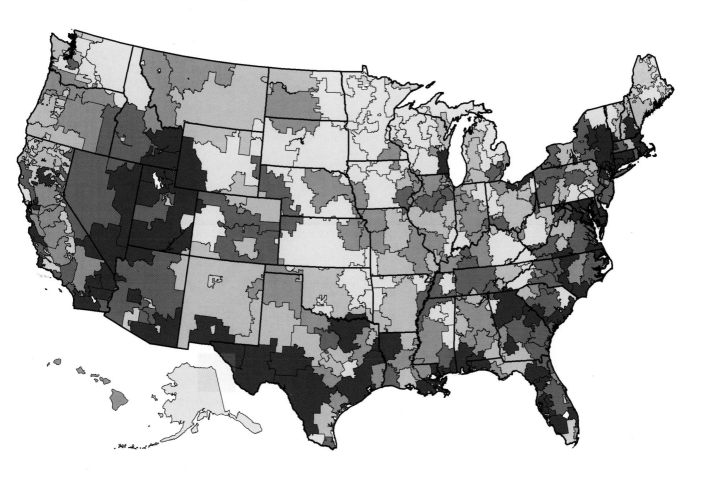

Map 5.a. The 50/50 Rule

Although the percentage of the physician workforce in specialty practice might be expected to be highest in urban and densely populated areas, in fact large parts of the United States that are rural, particularly in the Mountain West, had high proportions of specialists compared to primary care physicians. In contrast, some rural areas, including Alaska and New Hampshire, had relatively high proportions of physicians in primary care.

**Percentage of Physicians
Who Are Specialists**
by Hospital Referral Region (1993)

- 66.4 to 72.5% (60 HRRs)
- 64.8 to <66.4% (62)
- 63.4 to <64.8% (59)
- 61.4 to <63.4% (63)
- 53.4 to <61.4% (62)
- Not Populated

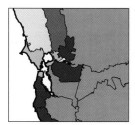

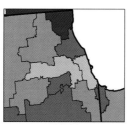

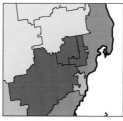

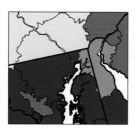

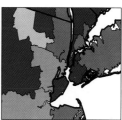

San Francisco   **Chicago**   **Detroit**   **Washington-Baltimore**   **New York**

For example, Wichita, Kansas, had a mix of specialists and primary care physicians in 1993 that was close to the proposed 50/50 goal. Wichita's supply of primary care physicians per hundred thousand residents (62.0) was close to the national average, but the city's supplies of specialists per hundred thousand residents (80.2) and of all physicians (142.9) were in the lowest fifth of all hospital referral regions. In contrast, although the physician workforce in White Plains, New York, had only about 31% generalists, the supply of generalists per hundred thousand residents in White Plains (93.7) was about 51% higher than the supply in Wichita. The proportion of generalists in White Plains was lower than in Wichita, but the per capita numbers of primary care physicians available to treat the local population were higher.

A comparison between Minneapolis and Dayton, Ohio, provides another example of the importance of examining the supply of physicians per hundred thousand residents instead of the proportion of generalists within an area. The proportion of the physician workforce in generalist practice in Minneapolis (41.3%) in 1993 was close to that in Dayton (38.8%), but the supply of generalist physicians per hundred thousand residents was 25% higher in Minneapolis (70.9) than in Dayton (56.9).

The Association Between the Primary Care and Specialist Physician Workforces and Medicare Reimbursements for Physicians' Services

The marked variation in the per capita supply of physicians across regions raises the question of whether spending for physician services is higher in areas with a greater physician supply. We examined correlations between Medicare spending for medical and surgical services and the supply of primary and specialty physicians.

There is a significant relationship between the specialist physician supply per hundred thousand residents and Medicare spending on physicians' services. As the supply of specialist physicians increases by 100 per hundred thousand population (e.g., from 150 to 250), Medicare spending could be predicted to increase by $136 per enrollee ($R^2 = .15$).

By contrast, the association between the capacity of the primary care physician workforce and Medicare reimbursements for medical and surgical services shows virtually no relationship between costs and reimbursements ($R^2 = .01$).

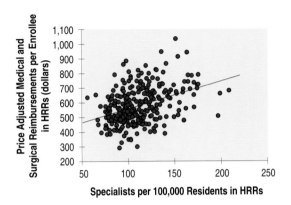

Figure 5.a. The Association Between the Specialty Physician Workforce and Price Adjusted Medicare Medical and Surgical Reimbursements (1993)

There was a significant but modest relationship between total physician supply per capita and Medicare spending on physicians' services. As the physician supply increases, Medicare spending could also be predicted to increase.

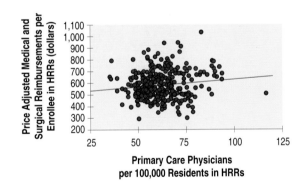

Figure 5.b. The Association Between the Primary Care Physician Workforce and Price Adjusted Medicare Medical and Surgical Reimbursements (1993)

There was virtually no association between the capacity of the primary care physician workforce and Medicare reimbursements for medical and surgical services.

Anesthesiologists

Between 1970 and 1993, the number of clinically active anesthesiologists rose more than 170%, from 8,942 to 24,469. The number of anesthesiologists per hundred thousand residents rose from 4.3 to 9.8, a factor of more than 2.25.

Although Hackensack, New Jersey, with 16.0 per hundred thousand population, was among the hospital referral regions with the highest ratio of anesthesiologists, there was a clear pattern of high anesthesiologist supply in the Mountain States and the West. Seattle (14.2), Salt Lake City (13.6), and Orange County, California (13.0), were typical of this trend.

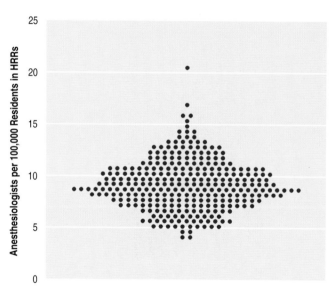

Among the regions with the lowest numbers of anesthesiologists per hundred thousand residents in 1993 were Charlotte, North Carolina (6.4); Wichita, Kansas (6.7); Omaha, Nebraska (7.3); and Birmingham, Alabama (7.5). Others that were below the national average were Ann Arbor, Michigan (8.0); Nashville, Tennessee (8.4); and Knoxville, Tennessee (8.0).

Figure 5.4. Anesthesiologists Allocated to Hospital Referral Regions (1993)

The number of anesthesiologists in active practice per hundred thousand residents, after adjusting for differences in age and sex of the local population, ranged from fewer than 4 to more than 20. Each point represents one of the 306 hospital referral regions in the United States.

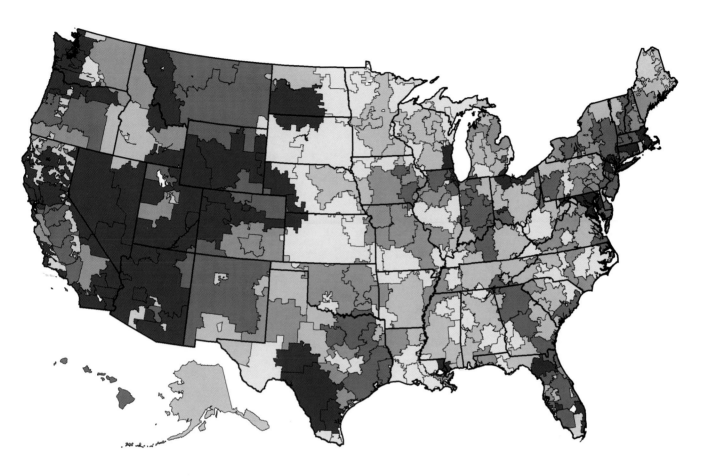

Map 5.4. Anesthesiologists

In 1993, the numbers of anesthesiologists per hundred thousand residents were high in the West, in parts of Texas, and on the West Coast; metropolitan areas also tended to have high supplies.

Anesthesiologists per 100,000 Residents

by Hospital Referral Region (1993)

- 11.05 to 20.43 (60 HRRs)
- 9.61 to <11.05 (61)
- 8.48 to < 9.61 (61)
- 7.23 to < 8.48 (62)
- 3.94 to < 7.23 (62)
- Not Populated

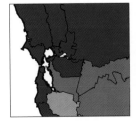

San Francisco

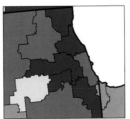

Chicago

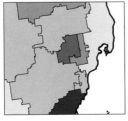

Detroit

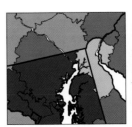

Washington-Baltimore

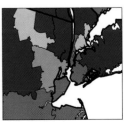

New York

Cardiologists

In 1970, there were 4,616 clinically active cardiologists practicing in the United States, or 2.2 for every hundred thousand residents. By 1993, the number of cardiologists had risen to 14,125, or 5.7 per hundred thousand residents. The actual number of cardiologists rose by a factor of 3.1, and the number per hundred thousand residents rose by a factor of 2.6.

Hospital referral regions with very high supplies of cardiologists in 1993 were heavily concentrated on the East Coast. Among the regions with the highest numbers of cardiologists per hundred thousand residents were Miami (10.1); Philadelphia (9.8); Hackensack, New Jersey (9.3); Manhattan (9.3); Washington, D.C. (9.2); and White Plains, New York (8.4).

Areas below the national average included Wichita, Kansas (3.5); Little Rock, Arkansas (3.9); Fort Worth, Texas (4.0); Charlotte, North Carolina (4.0); and Nashville, Tennessee (4.3).

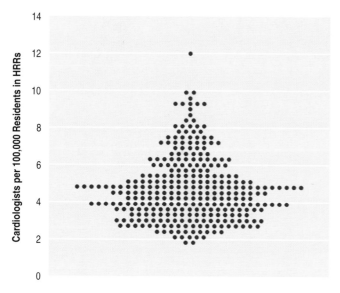

Figure 5.5. Cardiologists Allocated to Hospital Referral Regions (1993)

The number of cardiologists in active practice per hundred thousand residents, after adjusting for differences in age and sex of the local population, ranged from fewer than 2 to 12. Each point represents one of the 306 hospital referral regions in the United States.

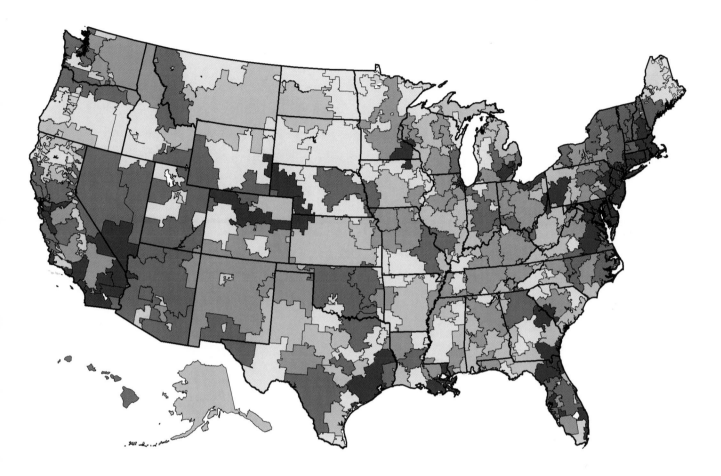

Map 5.5. Cardiologists

In 1993, the numbers of cardiologists per hundred thousand residents were
generally higher on the East and West Coasts, and lower in the Midwest
and parts of the South.

**Cardiologists
per 100,000 Residents**
by Hospital Referral Region (1993)

- 6.11 to 12.01 (62 HRRs)
- 4.80 to < 6.11 (61)
- 4.08 to < 4.80 (58)
- 3.29 to < 4.08 (62)
- 1.68 to < 3.29 (63)
- Not Populated

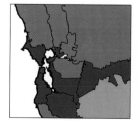

San Francisco

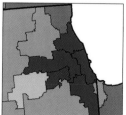

Chicago

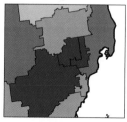

Detroit

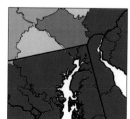

Washington-Baltimore

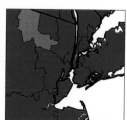

New York

General Surgeons

Between 1970 and 1993, the number of clinically active general surgeons in the United States rose from 22,204 to 24,060, an increase of only 8%, the smallest increase among specialists. The number of general surgeons per hundred thousand residents actually declined by about 10%, from 10.7 in 1970 to 9.7 in 1993.

Hospital referral regions with very high numbers of general surgeons per hundred thousand residents in 1993 included White Plains, New York (14.4); Baltimore (13.5); Buffalo, New York (12.9); Providence, Rhode Island (12.7); Washington, D.C. (12.6); and Hackensack, New Jersey (12.4). Manhattan (12.1) and East Long Island, New York (12.6), also had higher than average supplies of general surgeons.

Among the regions with numbers of general surgeons per hundred thousand residents below the national average in 1993 were Kansas City, Missouri (8.1); Orlando, Florida (8.2); Columbus, Ohio (8.2); Indianapolis (8.3); Tulsa, Oklahoma (8.4); San Bernardino, California (8.4); and Arlington, Virginia (8.5).

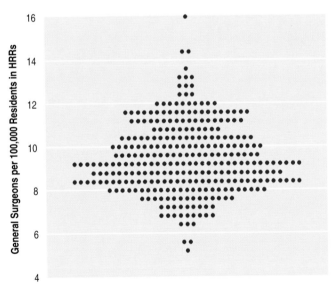

Figure 5.6. General Surgeons Allocated to Hospital Referral Regions (1993)

The number of general surgeons in active practice per hundred thousand residents, after adjusting for differences in age and sex of the local population, ranged from 5.3 to 16. Each point represents one of the 306 hospital referral regions in the United States.

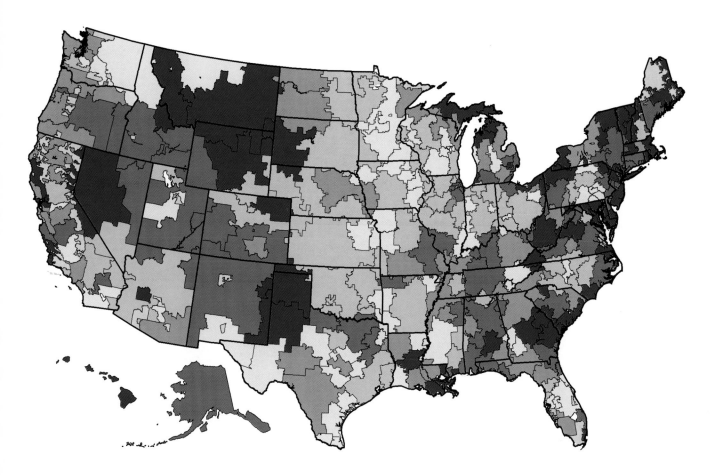

Map 5.6. General Surgeons

In 1993, the numbers of general surgeons per hundred thousand residents were highest on the East Coast and in the West, and lower throughout the Midwest.

General Surgeons per 100,000 Residents
by Hospital Referral Region (1993)

- 11.00 to 15.98 (61 HRRs)
- 9.73 to <11.00 (61)
- 8.87 to < 9.73 (60)
- 8.17 to < 8.87 (61)
- 5.26 to < 8.17 (63)
- Not Populated

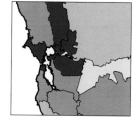

San Francisco

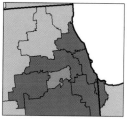

Chicago

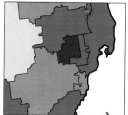

Detroit

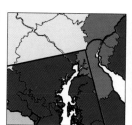

Washington-Baltimore

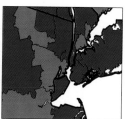

New York

Obstetrician/Gynecologists

In 1970, there were 15,460 obstetrician/gynecologists in active clinical practice in the United States; by 1993, there were 30,042, a 94% increase. The rate per hundred thousand residents increased by 62%, from 7.4 to 12.1.

Hospital referral regions with numbers of obstetrician/gynecologists per hundred thousand residents substantially above the national average in 1993 included White Plains, New York (19.7); East Long Island, New York (18.7); Fort Lauderdale, Florida (18.8); Hackensack, New Jersey (18.0); Baltimore (17.7); Washington, D.C. (17.5); and Camden, New Jersey (16.0).

Hospital referral regions with smaller populations were more heavily represented in the group of areas with low per capita supplies of obstetrician/gynecologists; among the lowest were Mason City, Iowa (6.8); La Crosse, Wisconsin (6.7); Grand Forks, North Dakota (6.5); Fort Wayne, Indiana (6.4); and Cedar Rapids, Iowa (6.1).

Few regions with populations of over one million residents had supplies below the national average. Among those large hospital referral regions which had relatively low numbers of obstetrician/gynecologists per hundred thousand residents in 1993 were Madison, Wisconsin (7.5); Wichita, Kansas (7.8); Des Moines, Iowa (7.9); Omaha, Nebraska (8.7); Indianapolis (9.2); Lexington, Kentucky (9.4); Fresno, California (9.9); and Spokane, Washington (10.1).

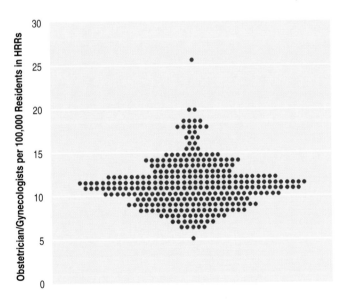

Figure 5.7. Obstetrician/Gynecologists Allocated to Hospital Referral Regions (1993)

The number of obstetrician/gynecologists in active practice per hundred thousand residents, after adjusting for differences in age and sex of the local population, ranged from 5.4 to more than 25. Each point represents one of the 306 hospital referral regions in the United States.

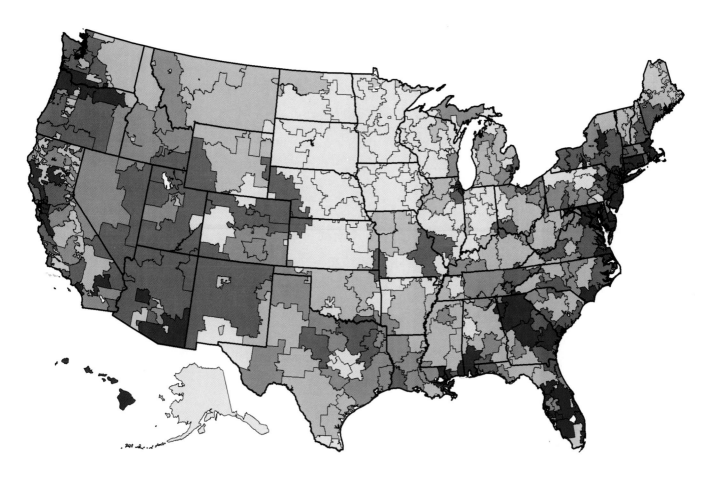

Map 5.7. Obstetrician/Gynecologists

In 1993, the numbers of obstetrician/gynecologists per hundred thousand residents were generally higher on the East and West Coasts than in the Midwest or the Mountain States.

Obstetrician/Gynecologists per 100,000 Residents
by Hospital Referral Region (1993)

- 13.25 to 25.65 (61 HRRs)
- 11.62 to <13.25 (61)
- 10.67 to <11.62 (61)
- 9.18 to <10.67 (60)
- 5.43 to < 9.18 (63)
- Not Populated

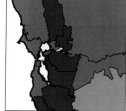

San Francisco

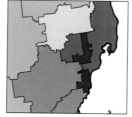

Chicago

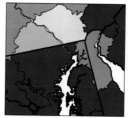

Detroit

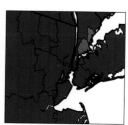

Washington-Baltimore

New York

Ophthalmologists

Between 1970 and 1993, the number of clinically active ophthalmologists practicing in the United States rose from 8,273 to 14,659, a 77% increase. The supply of ophthalmologists grew from 4.0 to 5.9 per hundred thousand residents of the country, an increase of 48%.

Among the hospital referral regions with high numbers of ophthalmologists per hundred thousand residents were White Plains, New York (10.9); Manhattan (8.5); and East Long Island, New York (8.7). Also well above the national average were Washington, D.C. (9.6); Hackensack, New Jersey (8.8); Miami (7.9); Baltimore (7.7); Honolulu (7.6); Denver (7.6); and New Haven, Connecticut (7.5).

The ophthalmologist workforces serving Wichita, Kansas (3.5); Charleston, West Virginia (4.0); Des Moines, Iowa (4.1); Winston-Salem, North Carolina (4.1); Knoxville, Tennessee (4.2); Springfield, Illinois (4.2); and Harrisburg, Pennsylvania (4.7), were well below the national average.

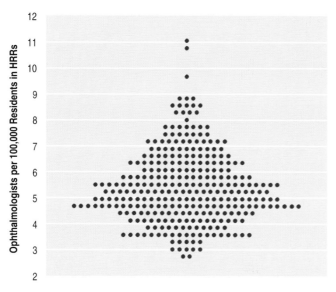

Figure 5.8. Ophthalmologists Allocated to Hospital Referral Regions (1993)

The number of ophthalmologists in active practice per hundred thousand residents, after adjusting for differences in age and sex of the local population, ranged from fewer than 3 to more than 11. Each point represents one of the 306 hospital referral regions in the United States.

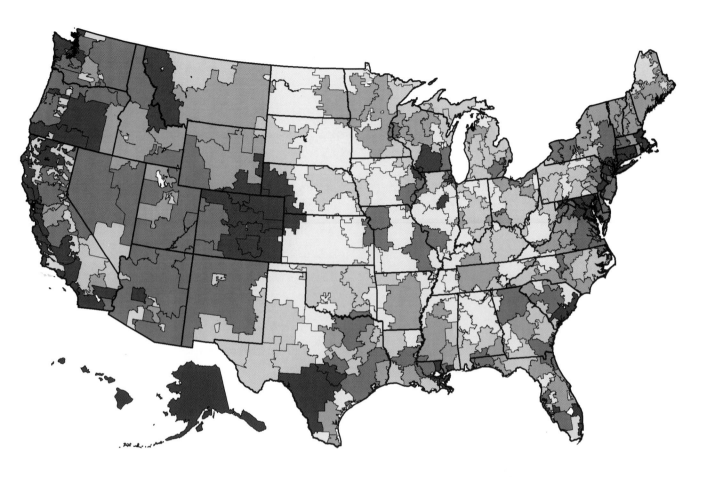

Map 5.8. Ophthalmologists

In 1993, the supply of ophthalmologists was higher on the East and West Coasts and in the West. The Midwest and the Ohio Valley generally had lower numbers of ophthalmologists per hundred thousand residents.

**Ophthalmologists
per 100,000 Residents**
by Hospital Referral Region (1993)

- 6.61 to 11.06 (62 HRRs)
- 5.58 to < 6.61 (58)
- 4.95 to < 5.58 (62)
- 4.33 to < 4.95 (61)
- 2.65 to < 4.33 (63)
- Not Populated

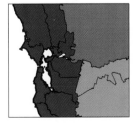

San Francisco

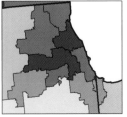

Chicago

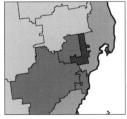

Detroit

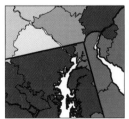

Washington-Baltimore

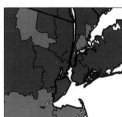

New York

Orthopedic Surgeons

In 1970, there were 7,537 clinically active orthopedic surgeons in the United States; by 1993, the number had increased more than 135% to 17,895. The number of orthopedic surgeons per hundred thousand residents doubled, from 3.6 to 7.2.

Among the hospital referral regions that had large populations, the highest numbers of orthopedic surgeons per hundred thousand residents in 1993 were in San Francisco (10.7); Seattle (10.2); Orange County, California (10.2); Portland, Maine (10.0); Fort Lauderdale, Florida (9.8); and San Diego (9.4).

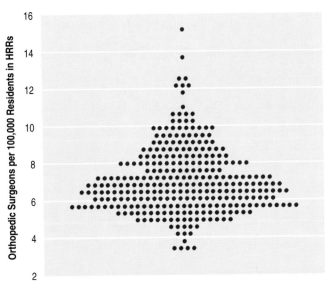

Hospital referral regions with the lowest numbers of orthopedic surgeons per hundred thousand residents in the United States in 1993 included the Bronx, New York (3.9); Memphis, Tennessee (4.7); Lexington, Kentucky (4.7); Ann Arbor, Michigan (4.9); and Springfield, Illinois (4.9).

Figure 5.9. Orthopedic Surgeons Allocated to Hospital Referral Regions (1993)

The number of orthopedic surgeons in active practice per hundred thousand residents, after adjusting for differences in age and sex of the local population, ranged from 3.2 to more than 15. Each point represents one of the 306 hospital referral regions in the United States.

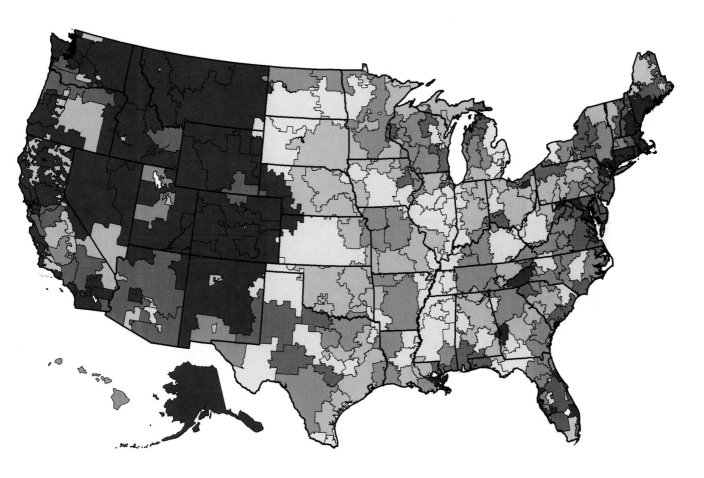

Map 5.9. Orthopedic Surgeons

In 1993, the numbers of orthopedic surgeons per hundred thousand residents tended to be far higher in the West, in Florida, and in parts of the Northeast; the numbers in the Midwest and South tended to be low.

Orthopedic Surgeons per 100,000 Residents
by Hospital Referral Region (1993)

- 8.53 to 15.19 (60 HRRs)
- 7.12 to < 8.53 (61)
- 6.39 to < 7.12 (62)
- 5.70 to < 6.39 (61)
- 3.23 to < 5.70 (62)
- Not Populated

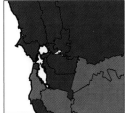

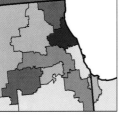

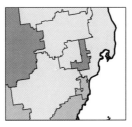

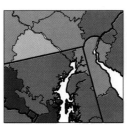

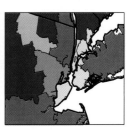

| San Francisco | Chicago | Detroit | Washington-Baltimore | New York |

Psychiatrists

The number of clinically active psychiatrists in the United States almost doubled between 1970 and 1993, from 16,450 to 32,254. The number per hundred thousand residents increased by 64%, from 7.9 to 13.0.

More than any other specialty, the number of psychiatrists per hundred thousand population tended to be highest in urban areas. Among the regions with the highest numbers of psychiatrists per hundred thousand residents in 1993 were White Plains, New York (43.9); San Francisco (38.4); Manhattan (35.5); East Long Island, New York (25.8); the Bronx, New York (24.5); Boston (30.5); Washington, D.C. (29.5); New Haven, Connecticut (25.2); Philadelphia (24.7); Hackensack, New Jersey (24.1); Hartford, Connecticut (22.3); and Lebanon, New Hampshire (22.1).

Most hospital referral regions that had very low numbers of psychiatrists per hundred thousand residents had relatively small populations (well under one million). Among these were Oxford, Mississippi (2.8); Fort Smith, Arkansas (3.0); Lake Charles, Louisiana (3.3); Paducah, Kentucky (3.4); and McAllen, Texas (3.4).

Larger areas with relatively low numbers of psychiatrists in 1993, compared to the national average, were Des Moines, Iowa (5.9); Birmingham, Alabama (6.4); Fort Worth, Texas (6.7); Wichita, Kansas (6.8); Tulsa, Oklahoma (7.0); Memphis, Tennessee (7.1); and El Paso, Texas (7.1).

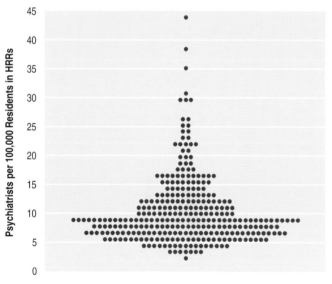

Figure 5.10. Psychiatrists Allocated to Hospital Referral Regions (1993)

The number of psychiatrists in active practice per hundred thousand residents, after adjusting for differences in age and sex of the local population, ranged from 2.5 to almost 44. Each point represents one of the 306 hospital referral regions in the United States.

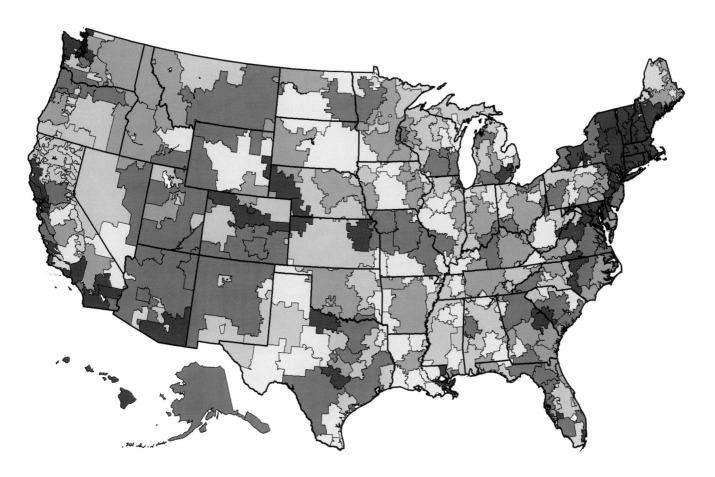

Map 5.10. Psychiatrists

In 1993, most major metropolitan areas and the East and West Coasts had much higher numbers of psychiatrists per hundred thousand residents than the Plains States, the Ohio Valley, and the South.

Psychiatrists per 100,000 Residents

by Hospital Referral Region (1993)

- 13.88 to 43.88 (61 HRRs)
- 9.73 to <13.88 (61)
- 7.85 to < 9.73 (61)
- 6.29 to < 7.85 (60)
- 2.51 to < 6.29 (63)
- Not Populated

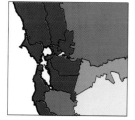

San Francisco

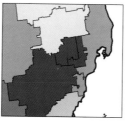

Chicago

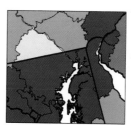

Detroit

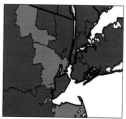

Washington-Baltimore

New York

Radiologists

There were 22,413 clinically active radiologists practicing in the United States in 1993, up 142% from the 1970 level of 9,245. The number of radiologists per hundred thousand residents more than doubled, rising from 4.4 to 9.0.

The number of radiologists per hundred thousand residents was about 30% higher than the national average in Philadelphia (13.6); White Plains, New York (13.4); Boston (13.0); Washington, D.C. (12.5); and Durham, North Carolina (12.1). Other areas with high rates in 1993 were Cleveland (12.0), Pittsburgh (11.8), Baltimore (11.3), and Seattle (11.0).

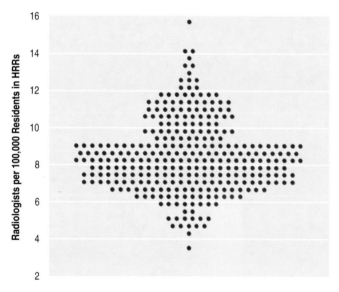

Hospital referral regions where the allocated workforce was less than the national average included El Paso, Texas (5.0); Austin, Texas (6.1); Columbus, Ohio (6.7); Grand Rapids, Michigan (6.9); Fort Worth, Texas (7.2); and San Bernardino, California (7.2).

Figure 5.11. Radiologists Allocated to Hospital Referral Regions (1993)

The number of radiologists in active practice per hundred thousand residents, after adjusting for differences in age and sex of the local population, ranged from 3.3 to 15.7. Each point represents one of the 306 hospital referral regions in the United States.

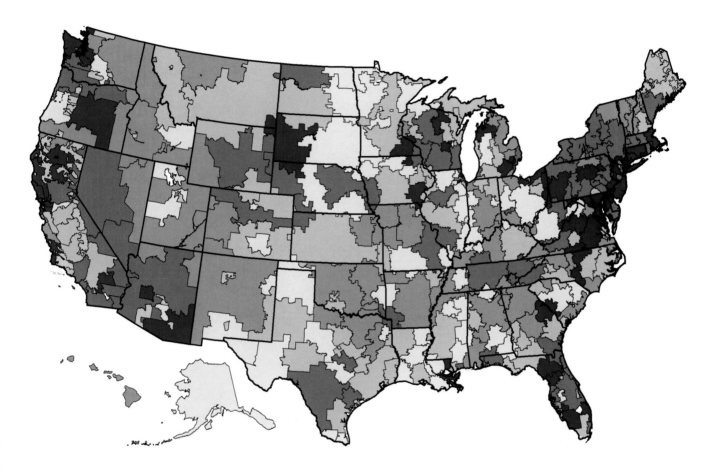

Map 5.11. Radiologists

In 1993, the numbers of radiologists per hundred thousand residents were high on the West Coast and in parts of Colorado, Nebraska, Kansas, Florida, and the Mid-Atlantic states.

**Radiologists
per 100,000 Residents**
by Hospital Referral Region (1993)

- 10.08 to 15.69 (60 HRRs)
- 8.71 to <10.08 (61)
- 7.92 to < 8.71 (60)
- 6.92 to < 7.92 (63)
- 3.33 to < 6.92 (62)
- Not Populated

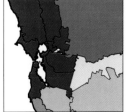

San Francisco

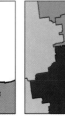
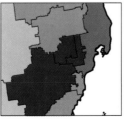

Chicago

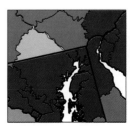

Detroit

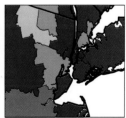

Washington-Baltimore

New York

Urologists

The number of urologists in active clinical practice in the United States grew 74% from 4,745 in 1970 to 8,246 in 1993 and the number of urologists per hundred thousand residents increased 46%, from 2.3 to 3.3.

Among the hospital referral regions with the highest numbers of urologists per hundred thousand residents were Washington, D.C. (5.0); White Plains, New York (4.9); Hackensack, New Jersey (4.5); Morristown, New Jersey (4.3); Newark, New Jersey (4.2); New Orleans (4.5); Miami (4.2); Fort Lauderdale, Florida (4.2); Seattle (4.1); Manhattan (4.1); and Atlanta (4.0).

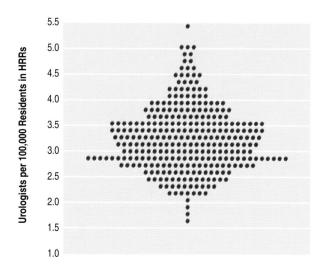

The workforces serving hospital referral regions in the Midwest tended to be relatively small; among the regions with low allocations per hundred thousand residents were Madison, Wisconsin (2.2); Fort Worth, Texas (2.3); Omaha, Nebraska (2.4); Detroit (2.5); and Wichita, Kansas (2.6). Portland, Maine (2.6); and Lebanon, New Hampshire (2.7), were among the East Coast hospital referral regions with relatively low supplies of urologists per hundred thousand residents.

Figure 5.12. Urologists Allocated to Hospital Referral Regions (1993)

The number of urologists in active practice per hundred thousand residents, after adjusting for differences in age and sex of the local population, ranged from 1.6 to 5.4. Each point represents one of the 306 hospital referral regions in the United States.

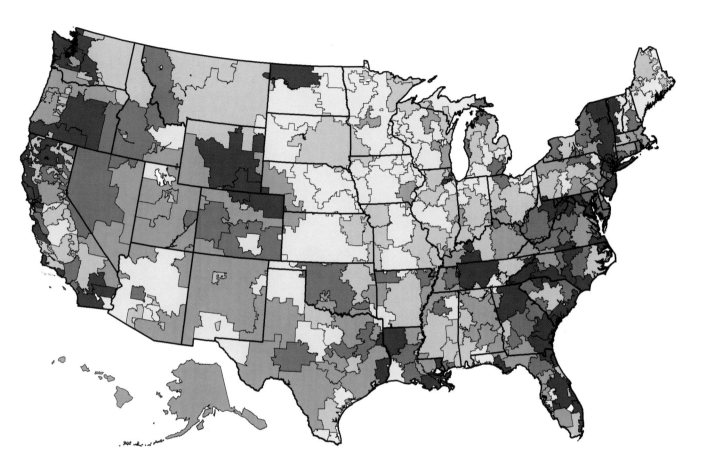

Map 5.12. Urologists

In 1993, the numbers of urologists per hundred thousand residents were high in some hospital referral regions in the Northeast and Mid-Atlantic states, in the Southeast, and along the West Coast. Most of the Midwest had relatively low supplies of urologists.

**Urologists
per 100,000 Residents**
by Hospital Referral Region (1993)

- 3.72 to 5.44 (63 HRRs)
- 3.34 to <3.72 (60)
- 3.02 to <3.34 (58)
- 2.75 to <3.02 (59)
- 1.61 to <2.75 (66)
- Not Populated

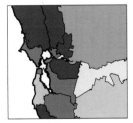

San Francisco

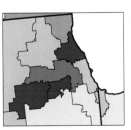

Chicago

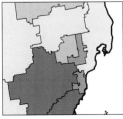

Detroit

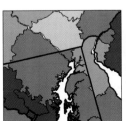

Washington-Baltimore

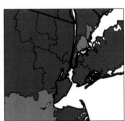

New York

Physicians in Residency Training Programs

In 1970, there were 52,233 physicians in residency training programs throughout the United States; by 1993, the numbers had increased 86%, to 97,047. The rate increased by 55%, from 25.1 to 39.0 per hundred thousand population. The distribution of resident physicians among hospital referral regions in 1993 was very uneven, ranging from 6.6 per hundred thousand residents in Billings, Montana, to 113.0 in Rochester, Minnesota.

Among the regions with the highest numbers of physicians in residency training programs per hundred thousand population were Rochester, Minnesota (113.0); Manhattan (111.1); Chicago (98.7); the Bronx, New York (97.6); Durham, North Carolina (87.4); Ann Arbor, Michigan (78.8); Philadelphia (77.8); Boston (77.1); New Orleans (76.7); Cleveland (70.8); Washington, D.C. (68.7); San Francisco (65.3); Detroit (61.4); and New Haven, Connecticut (61.0).

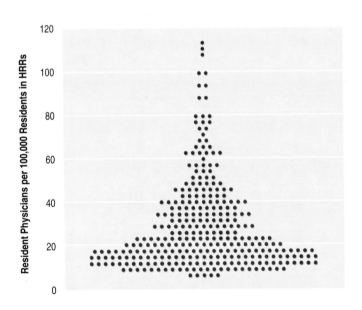

The hospital referral regions with the lowest numbers of physicians in residency training programs per hundred thousand population were those with populations of under one million. Larger referral regions that had fewer than 20 physicians in residency training programs per hundred thousand population in 1993 included Spokane, Washington (12.9); Orlando, Florida (15.0); Knoxville, Tennessee (15.5); Fort Worth, Texas (18.2); and Charlotte, North Carolina (18.7).

Figure 5.13. Physicians in Residency Training Programs Allocated to Hospital Referral Regions (1993)

The number of physicians in residency training programs per hundred thousand residents ranged from 6.6 to 113.0. Each point represents one of the 306 hospital referral regions in the United States.

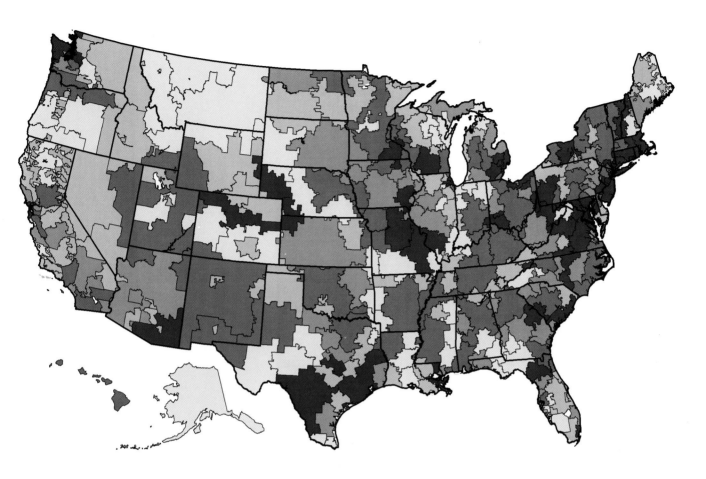

Map 5.13. Physicians in Residency Training Programs

In 1993, the highest numbers of physicians in residency training programs per hundred thousand population were in urban areas, most notably in the densely populated East Coast corridor. There were fewer, and smaller, training programs relative to the population size in more sparsely populated areas of the country, such as the Mountain States and Maine.

**Physicians in
Residency Training
per 100,000 Residents**
by Hospital Referral Region (1993)

- 41.55 to 113.00 (60 HRRs)
- 28.10 to <41.55 (62)
- 18.15 to <28.10 (60)
- 12.77 to <18.15 (61)
- 6.56 to <12.77 (63)
- Not Populated

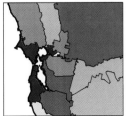

San Francisco

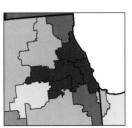

Chicago

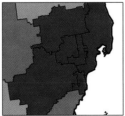

Detroit

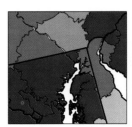

Washington-Baltimore

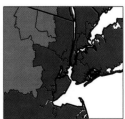

New York

PART SIX

The Diagnosis and Surgical Treatment of Common Medical Conditions

The Diagnosis and Surgical Treatment of Common Medical Conditions

Jacob Bigelow, in an 1835 address to the Massachusetts Medical Society, observed that "A man who falls sick at home or abroad is liable to get heroic treatment, or nominal treatment, random treatment, or no treatment at all, according to the hands into which he happens to fall."

Since Bigelow's time, doctors and researchers have continued to observe puzzling variations in rates of common surgical procedures among seemingly similar populations. In the 1930s, the British pediatrician J. Alison Glover noted that in some school districts more than half of the children had had tonsillectomies before they were 18, while in other districts fewer than 10% had had the surgery. Glover traced the variation to differences in professional opinion among school health officers about the usefulness of tonsillectomy in preventing illness. Some doctors believed that in order to avoid hearing loss and learning disability, tonsils should be removed at the slightest evidence of infection. Others believed that tonsils must serve some function and were reluctant to remove them unless infection became a serious problem, which it rarely did.

Although Glover identified disagreement among physicians as the source of variation, and even undertook outcome studies of children who had had tonsillectomies, it was not until well after the Second World War that clinical trials of "preventive" tonsillectomy versus "watchful waiting" (monitoring without surgical intervention) were undertaken. The results upheld Glover's conjecture that preventive tonsillectomy was not an effective strategy.

The Problem of Scientific Uncertainty

Failure to evaluate the outcomes of care makes it possible for different theories and opinions on the risks and benefits of alternative treatments to coexist, unchallenged by fact. In recent years, greater awareness of practice variations has increased public understanding of the need to conduct systematic studies of the outcomes of care. However, what has been referred to as a double standard of truth in medicine persists. While the Food and Drug Administration assures that new drugs are tested to determine that they have clinical efficacy before they are widely marketed, the outcomes of other treatment options, such as surgical procedures and medical devices (and drugs used in ways not tested prior to Food and Drug Administration approval), are not systematically subjected to evaluation. Until clinical research is applied uniformly to all treatment options, many good medical ideas will remain unproven and many strategies that do not work will remain in active use. Patients and physicians will continue to face unnecessary scientific uncertainty about the risks and benefits of care.

Which Surgical Rate Is Right?

Scientific uncertainty is not a sufficient explanation for practice variations. An answer to the question "Which rate is right?" depends on knowing who should decide. Unwanted variations in the use of diagnostic and surgical procedures are inevitable in clinical environments where the preferences of providers or managed care companies, rather than those of patients, dominate the choice of treatment.

The problem of unwanted variations in the rates of surgery thus has its origins in the traditional doctor-patient relationship – in the deep conviction that doctors know best. Since the time of Hippocrates, this tradition has held that the physician should make the decision about what treatment to use, based on his or her superior knowledge of what the patient wants. Since the Second World War, this model has been challenged, most significantly by the legal doctrine of informed consent, which demands that patients need to be fully informed about their options before consenting to the recommended treatment.

More recently, the challenge has been to the nature of the doctor-patient relationship itself. For many conditions, the extraordinary success of biomedical science and technology has created a rich range of diagnostic and therapeutic options. These options can have very different costs, risks, and benefits. Individual patients have different attitudes toward risks and different preferences for outcomes. Given the number of options, it is impossible for providers to accurately intuit how the individual patient would choose. To obtain the treatment they want, patients must evaluate the costs and benefits of treatment for themselves.

To find out which rate is right, patients must be informed about the options and must be free to choose according to their own preferences. This section of the Atlas provides a number of examples of practice variations that can only be remedied by bringing the patient into the clinical decision making process – by reforming the doctor-patient relationship to incorporate shared decision making.

Underservice

Variations can also reveal the failure of health care plans and providers to provide benefits that work and that most patients would want if they were informed about their value. A good example is mammography among women over the age of 50, which has been shown to reduce premature death from breast cancer. This section demonstrates significant underservice of mammography throughout the United States.

The Diagnosis and Treatment of Coronary Artery Disease

Chest pain due to blockage of the arteries that feed the heart (angina pectoris) is a common condition. Many patients with angina have several treatment options, including coronary artery bypass grafting (open heart surgery) and percutaneous transluminal coronary angioplasty (balloon angioplasty). Other approaches rely chiefly on the use of drugs to improve coronary artery flow; still others use strict dietary control of fat intake.

The pattern of variation in the use of angioplasty and bypass surgery from region to region provides important evidence about the existence of supplier-induced demand. First, the wide variation in rates among regions – with neighboring regions often showing strikingly different rates of intervention – suggests that patients' choices are not driving the variation; it is highly unlikely that the incidence of disease or patient preferences vary in such an idiosyncratic way.

Second, although bypass surgery and angioplasty are often alternative ways of treating the same condition, there is little evidence that one form of invasive treatment is being substituted for the other; many communities with high rates of bypass surgery also had high rates of angioplasty.

A third key factor driving the rate of use of invasive procedures is the supply of diagnostic technology. Coronary angiography is a diagnostic test that is an essential step in the discovery of coronary artery disease amenable to invasive treatment. Rates of coronary angiography were closely linked to the decision to undertake coronary artery bypass surgery or percutaneous transluminal coronary angioplasty. Medicare enrollees living in communities with higher per capita levels of diagnostic testing were much more likely to experience invasive treatments for coronary artery disease than those who lived in regions with relatively low testing rates.

Coronary Artery Bypass Grafting

Coronary artery bypass grafting (CABG) is a surgical procedure in which blood flow to the heart is rerouted through a substitute blood vessel. For some patients with angina, clinical trials have shown that CABG can prolong life; but most patients have forms of coronary artery disease for which the main benefit of treatment is reduction of pain or improved functional capacity. More than 300,000 CABG procedures were performed on Medicare enrollees over the age of 65 who had traditional Medicare coverage (that is, who were not enrolled in risk bearing health maintenance organizations) during 1992-93. The rates of CABG surgery per thousand Medicare enrollees varied by a factor of more than 4, from 2.1 in the Grand Junction, Colorado, hospital referral region, to 8.5 in the Joliet, Illinois, region.

Among the large hospital referral regions with the highest rates of CABG per thousand Medicare enrollees were Birmingham, Alabama (7.7); Memphis, Tennessee (7.7); Little Rock, Arkansas (7.1); and Dayton, Ohio (6.8). Hospital referral regions with more than one million residents that had low rates of the procedure included Albuquerque, New Mexico (2.7); Denver (3.1); Honolulu (3.4); and the Bronx, New York (3.5).

Lubbock, Texas, had a rate that was more than twice as high as Albuquerque, New Mexico, although the regions are contiguous; similarly, the Norfolk and Arlington hospital referral regions, both in Virginia, were at opposite ends of the spectrum. Rockford, Illinois, had a rate that was less than half that for the residents of nearby Joliet. The rate of bypass surgery in Saginaw, Michigan, was 60% higher than in Grand Rapids. The rate in Little Rock, Arkansas, was nearly 70% higher than in neighboring Jackson, Mississippi.

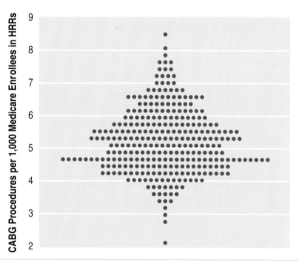

Figure 6.1. CABG Among Hospital Referral Regions (1992-93)

The number of CABG procedures varied from 2.1 to 8.5 per thousand Medicare enrollees, after adjusting for differences in age, sex, and race of the local population. Each point represents one of the 306 hospital referral regions in the United States.

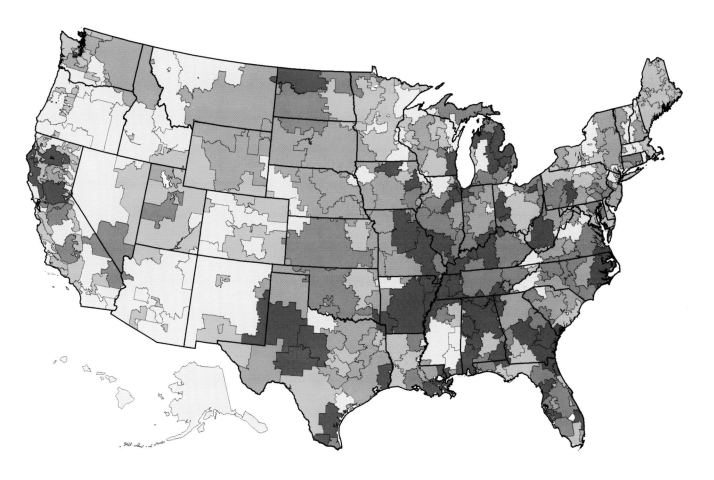

Map 6.1. Coronary Artery Bypass Grafting

Although rates tended to be lower in the West and Northeast in 1992-93, there were no strong geographic patterns; hospital referral regions with high rates were often near those where rates were low.

CABG Procedures per 1,000 Medicare Enrollees
by Hospital Referral Region (1992-93)

- 6.07 to 8.50 (62 HRRs)
- 5.40 to <6.07 (62)
- 4.86 to <5.40 (59)
- 4.43 to <4.86 (60)
- 2.06 to <4.43 (63)
- Not Populated

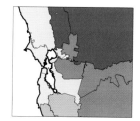

San Francisco

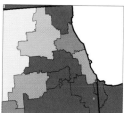

Chicago

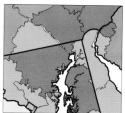

Detroit

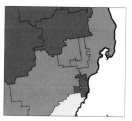

Washington-Baltimore

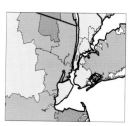

New York

Percutaneous Transluminal Coronary Angioplasty

Percutaneous transluminal coronary angioplasty (PTCA) is a procedure in which a catheter with a small balloon attached to it is inserted into the blocked artery; at the blockage, the balloon is inflated, pushing the fatty deposits against the artery wall. Angioplasty does not require open heart surgery, but its effects are usually less lasting than those of bypass grafts, and repeat procedures are required more often. More than 287,000 PTCA procedures were performed on Medicare enrollees over the age of 65 who had traditional Medicare coverage (that is, who were not enrolled in risk bearing health maintenance organizations) during 1992-93. The rate per thousand Medicare enrollees varied by a factor of 8, from 1.6 in Buffalo, New York, to 12.8 in Stockton, California.

Among the large hospital referral regions with high rates of PTCA per thousand Medicare enrollees were Milwaukee (8.1); Birmingham, Alabama (7.7); and Alameda County, California (7.4). Among the regions with the lowest rates of angioplasty, seven were in New York State. Other low rate regions included Lexington, Kentucky (2.8) and Albuquerque, New Mexico (2.9).

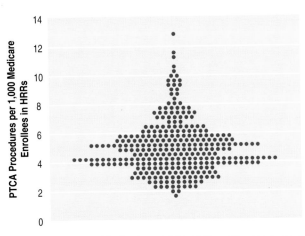

Figure 6.2. PTCA Among Hospital Referral Regions (1992-93)

The number of PTCA procedures performed varied from fewer than 2 to almost 13 per thousand Medicare enrollees, after adjusting for differences in age, sex, and race of the local population. Each point represents one of the 306 hospital referral regions in the United States.

In a few regions, there was an inverse relationship between PTCA and CABG; for example, in Texarkana, Arkansas, and Bloomington, Illinois, rates of CABG were high and rates of PTCA were relatively low. In Missoula, Montana, the PTCA rate was high while the CABG rate was low. Across the nation, however, the rates of the two procedures were positively correlated (R^2=.10). For example, rates for both CABG and PTCA were high in Birmingham, Alabama, and Milwaukee. In Albuquerque, New Mexico, and Syracuse, New York, the rates were low for both.

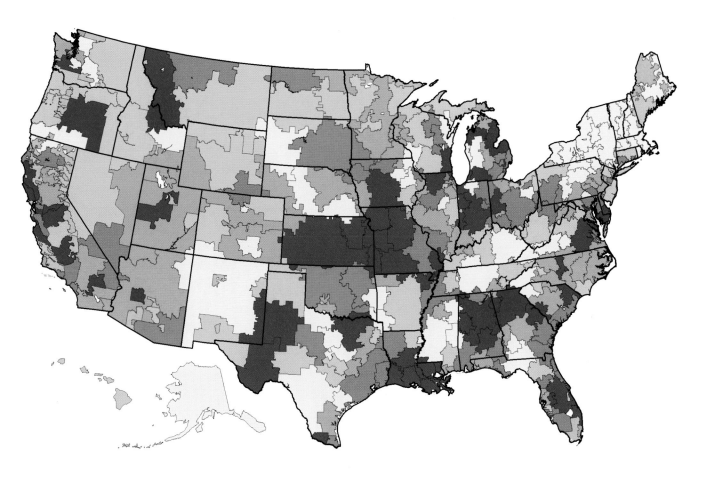

Map 6.2. Percutaneous Transluminal Coronary Angioplasty

The use of PTCA was variable within regions, and in some cases within states, in 1992-93. Rates were high in Kansas and neighboring parts of Missouri, but low in contiguous Nebraska. Rates were low in New York and most of New England, New Mexico, and parts of Kentucky and Tennessee. Within states, high rate areas often bordered low rate areas; Texas provides several examples.

PTCA Procedures per 1,000 Medicare Enrollees
by Hospital Referral Region (1992-93)

■	6.05 to 12.77 (63 HRRs)
■	5.10 to <6.05 (61)
■	4.23 to <5.10 (59)
■	3.62 to <4.23 (60)
□	1.63 to <3.62 (63)
■	Not Populated

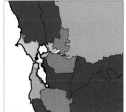

San Francisco

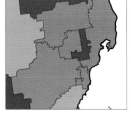

Chicago

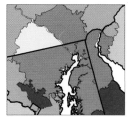

Detroit

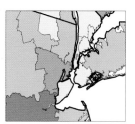

Washington-Baltimore

New York

Coronary Angiography

Coronary angiography is a diagnostic procedure in which contrast dye material is injected into the coronary arteries, making it possible to use imaging techniques to diagnose blockages in the blood vessels feeding the heart. More than 950,000 coronary angiography procedures were performed on Medicare enrollees over the age of 65 who had traditional Medicare coverage (that is, who were not enrolled in risk bearing health maintenance organizations) during 1993. The rate of coronary angiography per thousand Medicare enrollees varied by a factor of more than 4.7, from Waco, Texas (7.9), to Houma, Louisiana (37.5).

Among the hospital referral regions with rates of coronary angiography higher than 25 per thousand were Lubbock, Texas (31.8); Munster, Indiana (27.4); Rome, Georgia (27.4); Montgomery, Alabama (26.5); and Mobile, Alabama (25.7). Among regions with fewer than 10 procedures per thousand in 1992-93 were Honolulu (8.2); Lebanon, New Hampshire (8.2); Green Bay, Wisconsin (9.5); Muskegon, Michigan (9.7); and Medford, Oregon (9.9).

Coronary angiography is an essential diagnostic step in the decision making process leading to the recommendation of CABG or PTCA. There was a strong association between the rates of coronary angiography and the rates of these invasive treatments (R^2=.64).

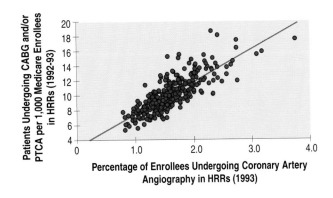

Figure 6.3. The Association Between the Incidence of Angiography (1993) and the Rates of CABG and PTCA (1992-93)

The number of Medicare enrollees undergoing one or more cardiac angiograms per thousand enrollees was closely linked to the combined rates of PTCA and CABG.

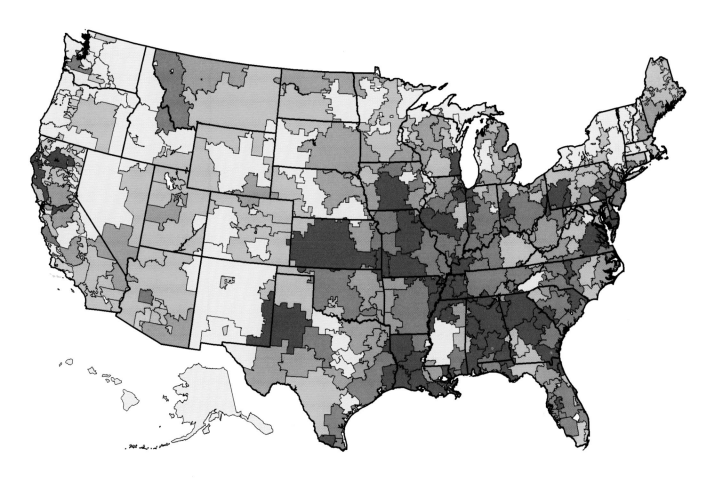

Map 6.3. Coronary Angiography

Coronary angiography rates were generally higher in the Eastern half of the United States than in the West. The exceptions were Northern California, where some areas had high rates, and the Northeast, where rates were relatively low, in 1993.

**Coronary Angiography
Procedures
per 1,000 Medicare Enrollees**
by Hospital Referral Region

- 19.3 to 37.5 (61 HRRs)
- 16.6 to <19.3 (61)
- 14.9 to <16.6 (61)
- 12.9 to <14.9 (61)
- 7.9 to <12.9 (62)
- Not Populated

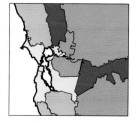

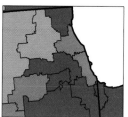

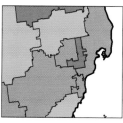

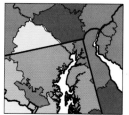

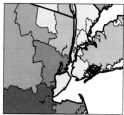

| San Francisco | Chicago | Detroit | Washington-Baltimore | New York |

The Diagnosis and Treatment of Breast Cancer

There is good evidence, based on numerous randomized clinical trials, about the efficacy of diagnostic screening and active treatment for improving health outcomes for breast cancer in women over the age of 50. Periodic mammograms for women in this age group result in a reduction of at least 30% in premature mortality from breast cancer.

Despite this evidence, and the consensus within the medical community that annual or biennial screening mammography should be routinely and uniformly offered to women over 50, there were wide variations in the rates at which women in the Medicare program actually had mammograms during 1992-93.

Different treatment options are available to women whose breast cancer has not spread beyond their breasts, including breast sparing surgery (partial mastectomy or lumpectomy) or excision of the entire breast (complete mastectomy). Breast sparing surgery, which involves the removal of only part of the breast, either the tissue immediately surrounding the tumor (lumpectomy) or a larger portion (partial mastectomy), reduces the disfigurement associated with total mastectomy. Clinical trials have shown little difference in death rates among women whose disease has not spread beyond the breast at the time of treatment, whether they undergo breast sparing surgery followed by radiation or chemotherapy, or whether they have total mastectomy.

The choice of treatment should depend on how individual women evaluate the risks and benefits of their choices, including how women feel about keeping their breasts; how they feel about radiation therapy and the risk of recurrence, should they choose partial mastectomy; and the issues of breast reconstruction or wearing a prosthesis, if they elect complete mastectomy. The pattern of variation, however, suggests that Medicare patients are not uniformly being advised about their options in ways that encourage them to participate in the decision making process.

Mammography

Mammography is a radiological examination of breast tissue, which, in women over the age of 50, is highly effective in identifying cancers of the breast. During 1993, about 3.6 million female Medicare enrollees over the age of 65 who had traditional Medicare coverage (that is, who were not enrolled in risk bearing health maintenance organizations), representing 20% of women in this category, had one or more mammograms. The percentage of all women enrolled in traditional Medicare on whom the examination was performed varied by a factor of more than 3.5 between regions, from Odessa, Texas (9.2%), to Sun City, Arizona (35.6%).

The percentage of female Medicare enrollees who had one or more mammograms was high, relative to the national average, in some hospital referral regions, including Lansing, Michigan (34.7%); Flint, Michigan (34.5%); Fort Lauderdale, Florida (34.2%); and Sarasota, Florida (33.8%). Rates of mammography in these regions were about three times higher than in low rate areas, but still fall far below the goal of an annual mammogram for women over 50.

The percentage female Medicare enrollees who had one or more mammorgrams was notably low in Oklahoma City (13.1%); Salt Lake City (13.4%); Memphis, Tennessee (13.9%); Albuquerque, New Mexico (14.2%); Fort Worth, Texas (14.3%); and Dallas (14.5%).

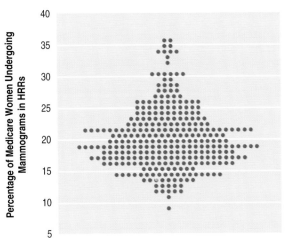

Figure 6.4. Mammography for Medicare Eligible Women Among Hospital Referral Regions (1993)

The percentage of women who had mammograms varied from about 9% to more than 35% of women enrolled in traditional Medicare, after adjusting for differences in age and race of the local population. Each point represents one of the 306 hospital referral regions in the United States.

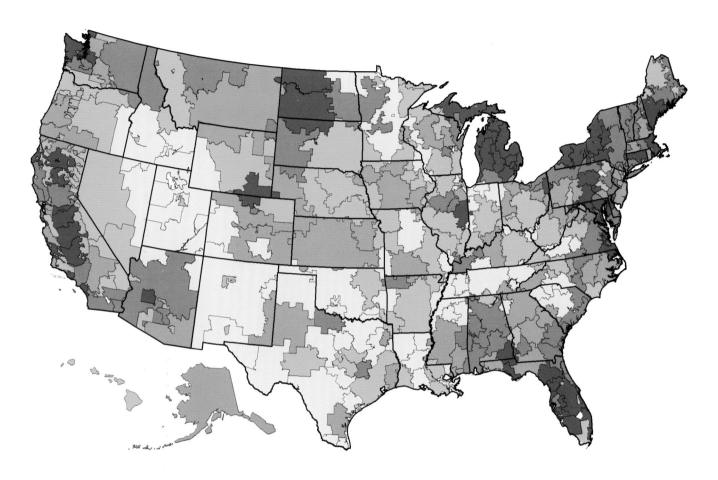

Map 6.4. Mammography

In 1993, the percentage of women undergoing one or more mammograms was high in the Northeast – notably New York State – and in Florida, Michigan, and most of California. North and South Dakota were remarkably split between high and low rate areas, as were Illinois, Colorado, and Wyoming.

Percentage of Medicare Women Who Had Mammograms
by Hospital Referral Region (1993)

- 24.1 to 35.6% (61 HRRs)
- 20.8 to <24.1% (61)
- 18.4 to <20.8% (61)
- 16.2 to <18.4% (61)
- 9.2 to <16.2% (62)
- Not Populated

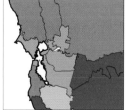

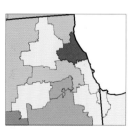

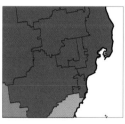

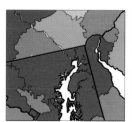

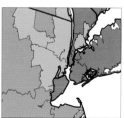

| San Francisco | Chicago | Detroit | Washington-Baltimore | New York |

Breast Sparing Surgery

Breast sparing surgery for breast cancer involves the removal of only part of the breast, either the tissue immediately surrounding the tumor (lumpectomy) or a larger portion (partial mastectomy). In 1992-93, more than 100,000 breast surgeries were performed on women over age 65 who were enrolled in traditional Medicare (that is, who were not enrolled in risk bearing health maintenance organizations) who were diagnosed with breast cancer. In spite of the evidence that there is little difference in survival rates between women who undergo partial mastectomy followed by chemotherapy or radiation, and women who have total mastectomies, the proportion of women who had breast sparing surgery varied by a factor of 33, from 1.4% of breast surgeries for cancer in Rapid City, South Dakota, to 48.0% in Elyria, Ohio.

Among the large hospital referral regions where the proportion of breast sparing surgery among women having surgery for breast cancer was over 30% were Paterson, New Jersey (37.8%); Ridgewood, New Jersey (34.8%); Boston (31.7%); Philadelphia (30.6%); East Long Island, New York (30.4%); and White Plains, New York (30.1%). Hospital referral regions in which the proportion of breast sparing surgery was under 5% included Ogden, Utah (1.9%); Yakima, Washington (3.8%); Fort Smith, Arkansas (4.3%); Fort Collins, Colorado (4.7%); and Joplin, Missouri (4.9%).

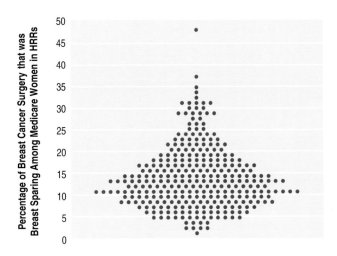

Figure 6.5. Use of Inpatient Breast Sparing Surgery for Medicare Eligible Women Among Hospital Referral Regions (1992-93)

The proportion of mastectomies for breast cancer that were breast sparing varied from 1.4% to 48.0%, after adjusting for age and race of the local population. Each point represents one of the 306 hospital referral regions in the United States.

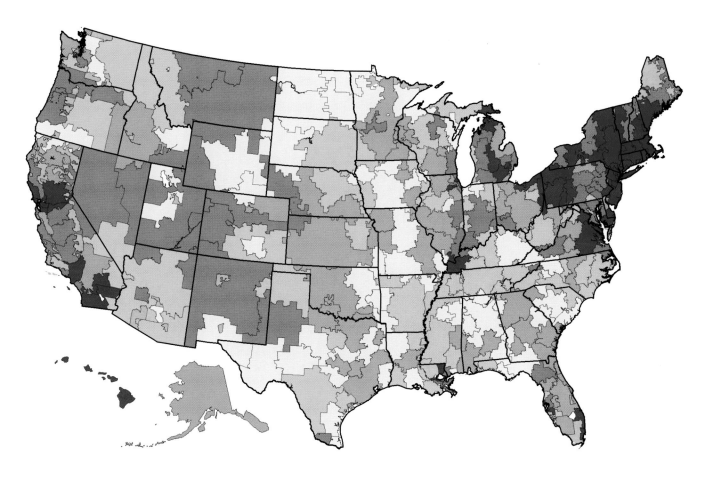

Map 6.5. Breast Sparing Surgery

Breast sparing surgery was more widely and commonly used in the Northeast than elsewhere in the United States; regionally, its use was lowest in the South, Midwest, and Northwest.

Percentage of Inpatient Breast Cancer Surgery in Medicare Women That Was Breast Sparing

by Hospital Referral Region (1992-93)

- 19.4 to 48.0% (61 HRRs)
- 14.5 to <19.4% (60)
- 11.3 to <14.5% (62)
- 8.1 to <11.3% (59)
- 1.4 to < 8.1% (64)
- Not Populated

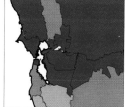

San Francisco

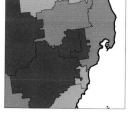

Chicago

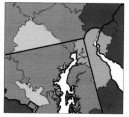

Detroit

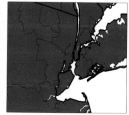

Washington-Baltimore

New York

The Treatment of Back Pain Due to Disc Disease

There are several strategies for dealing with back pain and related problems caused by injury to the intervertebral disc. Watchful waiting – monitoring the situation without surgical intervention – can lead to a cure if care is taken not to reinjure the spine. Exercise and medication are effective remedies for some patients, and this approach also avoids the risks and discomfort of surgery. Surgery does offer many patients a more rapid recovery, but carries with it a small but not insignificant risk that the effort to make things better may actually make them worse.

Patients with similar "objective" measures of disease experience the discomforts associated with disc injury differently. Some are very bothered by their condition, and wish to have surgery in the hope that it will offer a quicker and more definitive cure for their pain and loss of function; others with equally severe injury – as measured by examination of the spine – are not bothered enough by their symptoms to wish to undertake the discomforts and risks of surgery.

The patient's choice whether or not to undergo back surgery should depend most upon how the patient evaluates the risks and benefits of the available options. But as with other common conditions, the pattern of variation suggests that the decision to undergo back surgery is more likely to be driven by the physician's preference than the patient's.

Back Surgery

Back surgery is used to deal with pain and loss of mobility that may be caused by compression of the spinal canal or herniated vertebral discs. In 1992-93, more than 157,000 back surgery procedures were performed on Medicare enrollees over the age of 65 who had traditional Medicare coverage (that is, who were not enrolled in risk bearing health maintenance organizations). The rate of back surgery per thousand Medicare enrollees varied by a factor of almost 7, from 1.1 per thousand Medicare enrollees in Kingsport, Tennessee, to 7.0 per thousand in Provo, Utah.

Among the regions with the highest rates of back surgery per thousand Medicare enrollees were Fort Myers, Florida (5.5); Portland, Oregon (4.4); San Diego (4.1); Salt Lake City (4.0); and Tucson, Arizona (4.0). Regions that had relatively low rates of back surgery per thousand Medicare enrollees included the Bronx, New York (1.1); Manhattan (1.2); East Long Island, New York (1.2); Honolulu (1.4); and Miami (1.4).

The rates of back surgery in the Northeast as far south as Philadelphia (2.0) were among the lowest in the country; but the rate in Philadelphia's neighboring hospital referral region, Lancaster, Pennsylvania (4.3), was more than twice as high as in Philadelphia. Extremes were also seen in Florida: Miami (1.4) had the eighth lowest rate in the nation, while Fort Myers (5.5) was fifth from the top.

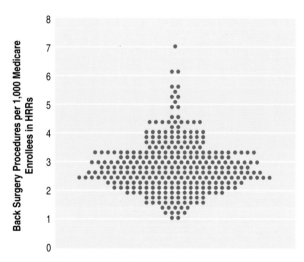

Figure 6.6. Back Surgery Among Hospital Referral Regions (1992-93)

The number of back surgery procedures per thousand Medicare enrollees, after adjusting for differences in age, sex, and race of the local population, ranged from 1.1 to 7.0. Each point represents one of the 306 hospital referral regions in the United States.

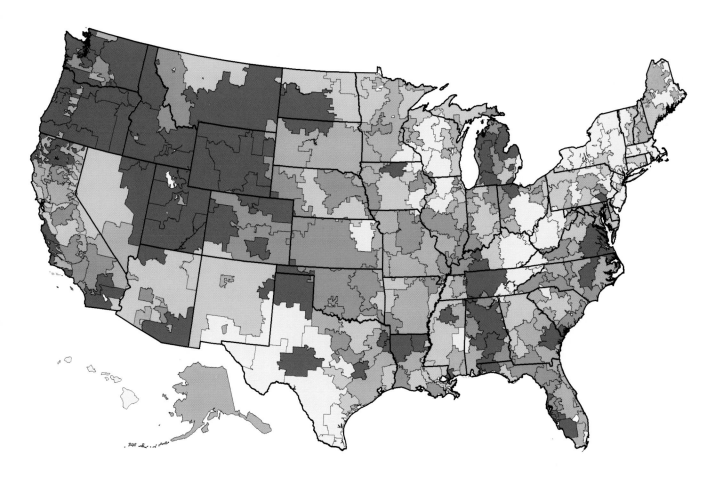

Map 6.6. Back Surgery

The rates of back surgery were much higher in the Mountain States and the
Northwest than in the Northeast or Upper Midwest in 1992-93.

**Back Surgery per 1,000
Medicare Enrollees**
by Hospital Referral Region
(1992-93)

- 3.44 to 7.02 (63 HRRs)
- 2.94 to <3.44 (61)
- 2.57 to <2.94 (57)
- 2.15 to <2.57 (63)
- 1.12 to <2.15 (62)
- Not Populated

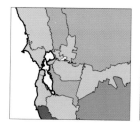

San Francisco

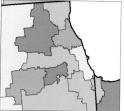

Chicago

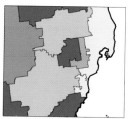

Detroit

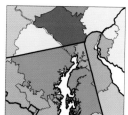

Washington-Baltimore

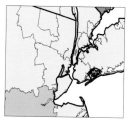

New York

The Diagnosis and Treatment of Early Stage Prostate Cancer

In recent years, the incidence of prostate biopsy has skyrocketed. The increase in biopsy rates is the result of a concerted effort in some areas to detect preclinical cancer with the prostate-specific antigen, or PSA, test. It is likely that the remarkable differences in biopsy rates from region to region are a reflection of the differences in the rates of PSA testing in those areas.

The controversy concerns not the test's ability to find early stage cancer, but the uncertainty about whether active treatment – surgery or radiation therapy – actually extends life expectancy. Unlike the case with many other forms of cancer, clinical trials to test the efficacy of treatment of early stage prostate cancer have not been completed. Untreated prostate cancer is usually slow growing and in most men does not become a clinical problem. For those men who have prostate cancer that is destined to cause problems, it is not clear that early treatment will significantly alter the course of events. The complications of treatment can be avoided by watchful waiting, or monitoring the situation without intervening.

Although science is uncertain about the outcomes, many physicians are quite certain about the treatment they prefer; and in the United States, preference generally reflects the physician's specialty. A 1988 study of physician preferences for the management of localized prostate cancer found that 79% of urologists in the United States recommended radical surgery, while 92% of radiation oncologists recommended radiation treatment. The large observed variations across the United States in both rates of prostate biopsy and rates of radical prostatectomy make a compelling case for the argument that physicians' choices, rather than those of patients, are driving the demand for the diagnosis and treatment of prostate cancer.

Prostate Biopsy

Prostate biopsy is a procedure in which a needle is inserted into the prostate gland to remove a small amount of tissue for microscopic study to determine the presence of cancer. More than 298,000 male Medicare enrollees over the age of 65, or 2.5% of all men who had traditional Medicare coverage (that is, who were not enrolled in risk bearing health maintenance organizations), had one or more prostate biopsies during 1993. The percentage of men undergoing prostate biopsy varied by a factor of 7, from Lafayette, Indiana (0.7%), to Houma, Louisiana (4.9%).

Among the hospital referral regions with high rates of prostate biopsy per thousand male Medicare enrollees in 1993 were Royal Oak, Michigan (4.7%); Pontiac, Michigan (4.6%); Dearborn, Michigan (4.4%); Orlando, Florida (4.0%); Las Vegas (4.0%); and Morristown, New Jersey (4.0%).

Among the regions where the rates of prostate biopsy per thousand male Medicare enrollees were low were Alameda County, California (1.4%); Chattanooga, Tennessee (1.6%); Greenville, North Carolina (1.7%); and Chicago (1.7%).

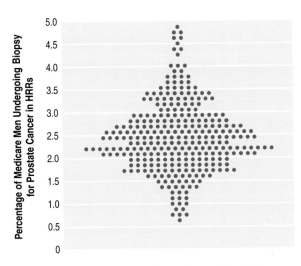

Figure 6.7. Prostate Biopsy Among Hospital Referral Regions (1993)

The percentage of men undergoing prostate biopsies varied from 0.7% to almost 5% of male Medicare enrollees, after adjusting for differences in age and race of the local population. Each point represents one of the 306 hospital referral regions in the United States.

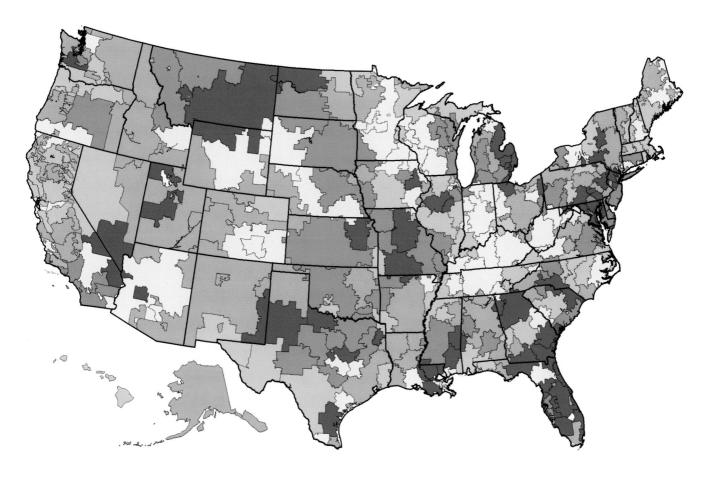

Map 6.7. Prostate Biopsy

There were no clear regional patterns in prostate biopsy rates; throughout the United States, high and low rate regions were juxtaposed. The rates were notably low in the Northeast and high in Montana and most of Florida; but in most parts of the country there were both high and low rate hospital referral regions.

Percentage of Medicare Men Who Had Prostate Biopsies
by Hospital Referral Region (1993)

- 3.01 to 4.87% (62 HRRs)
- 2.53 to <3.01% (63)
- 2.20 to <2.53% (57)
- 1.87 to <2.20% (59)
- 0.66 to <1.87% (65)
- Not Populated

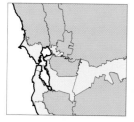

San Francisco

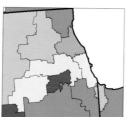

Chicago

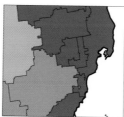

Detroit

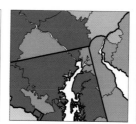

Washington-Baltimore

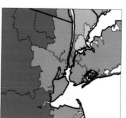

New York

Radical Prostatectomy

Radical prostatectomy is the complete surgical removal of the prostate gland. More than 65,000 radical prostatectomies were performed on Medicare enrollees over the age of 65 who had traditional Medicare coverage (that is, who were not enrolled in risk bearing health maintenance organizations) during 1992-93. The rates of radical prostatectomy varied by a factor of more than 4, from fewer than 1.5 per thousand in Lafayette, Louisiana; Providence, Rhode Island; and Chicago, to more than 6 per thousand in Palm Springs, California; Provo, Utah; and Boulder, Colorado.

Among the large hospital referral regions with high rates of radical prostatectomy per thousand male Medicare enrollees were Salt Lake City (5.6); Fresno, California (5.0); St. Paul, Minnesota (5.0); St. Louis (4.8); and Oklahoma City (4.7). Regions with comparatively low rates of radical prostatectomy included Manhattan (1.2); Camden, New Jersey (1.4); New Haven, Connecticut (1.5); and Louisville, Kentucky (1.5).

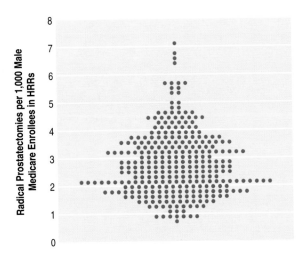

Figure 6.8. Radical Prostatectomy Among Hospital Referral Regions (1992-93)

The number of prostatectomies per thousand male Medicare enrollees varied from 0.6 to more than 7.0, after adjusting for differences in the age and race of the local population. Each point represents one of the 306 hospital referral regions in the United States.

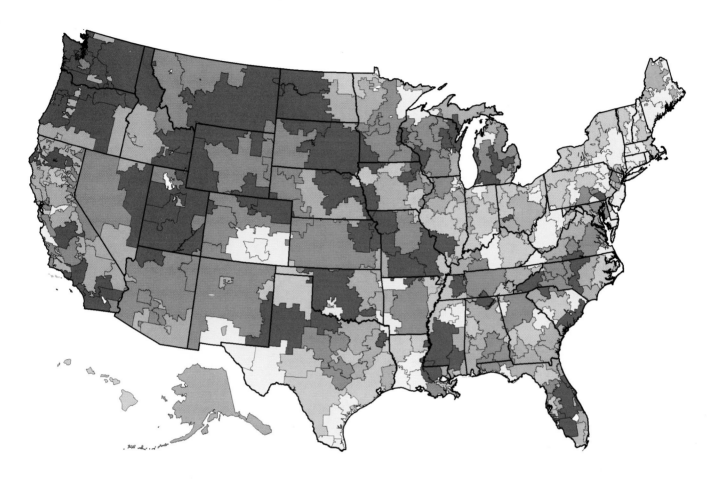

Map 6.8. Radical Prostatectomy

Rates of radical prostatectomy tended to be high in the Northwest, the Rocky Mountain States, and the Upper Midwest in 1992-93. Most sections of the country, with the exception of the Northeast, contain high rate regions. High rate regions are often contiguous with low rate regions: Texas, South Carolina, Pennsylvania, North Dakota, and California are examples.

Radical Prostatectomies per 1,000 Male Medicare Enrollees
by Hospital Referral Region (1992-93)

- ■ 3.68 to 7.11 (62 HRRs)
- ■ 3.02 to <3.68 (59)
- ■ 2.36 to <3.02 (62)
- ■ 1.82 to <2.36 (61)
- ■ 0.64 to <1.82 (62)
- ■ Not Populated

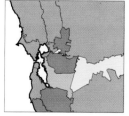

San Francisco

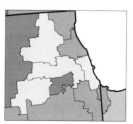

Chicago

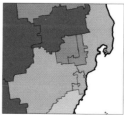

Detroit

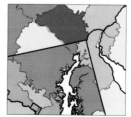

Washington-Baltimore

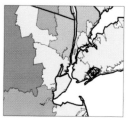

New York

The Diagnosis and Treatment of Benign Prostatic Hyperplasia

Benign prostatic hyperplasia (BPH) is a common condition affecting the majority of men over the age of 65. As men grow older, the prostate gland, which is near the outlet of the urinary bladder, often enlarges and causes urinary symptoms that some men find quite bothersome. The condition can be treated in several ways, including transurethral resection (surgical removal) of the prostate, other forms of surgery, medications, and watchful waiting. Surgery is effective in reducing symptoms for most men, and medications work well for some. The course of untreated BPH is variable.

Research conducted in the 1980s into the causes of the variations in surgery rates for BPH led to an important set of conclusions. Reducing unwanted variations in the patterns of practice required the active participation of the patient in the decision process, because the choice among treatments should depend on how individual patients assess the costs, risks, and benefits of the treatment options. For most men with BPH, the primary reasons for undergoing surgery are to reduce the severity of prostate-related symptoms and to improve the quality of life. The other approaches offer less improvement in symptoms but are also less risky. To make a rational choice among the options, the individual patient must assess his own situation, evaluating how much he is bothered by his symptoms and how concerned he is about possible adverse effects of active treatment.

Research has shown that when they are fully informed, most men with mild symptoms choose watchful waiting. Even though surgery is the most effective treatment for reducing symptoms, many men with moderate or severe symptoms prefer to live with their symptoms or accept less effective treatment to avoid the risk of surgery. Others accept the risk, willingly undergoing surgery because they are sufficiently bothered by their symptoms to want the benefits surgery offers.

Transurethral Resection of the Prostate for Benign Prostatic Hyperplasia

Transurethral resection of the prostate (TURP) is a surgical procedure in which part of the enlarged prostate is removed. More than 306,000 TURPs were performed on male Medicare enrollees over the age of 65 with a diagnosis of BPH who had traditional Medicare coverage (that is, who were not enrolled in risk bearing health maintenance organizations) during 1992-93. The number of TURPs per thousand male enrollees varied by a factor of more than 4, from 5.8 in Bryan, Texas, to 23.7 in Owensboro, Kentucky.

Among hospital referral regions with high rates per thousand men enrolled in traditional Medicare were Minot, North Dakota (19.7); Columbus, Georgia (19.6); Bend, Oregon (19.5); and Duluth, Minnesota (19.4). High rate regions with more than one million residents included Newark, New Jersey (17.9); Hackensack, New Jersey (17.4); Allentown, Pennsylvania (16.6); Wichita, Kansas (16.5); and Baltimore (15.9).

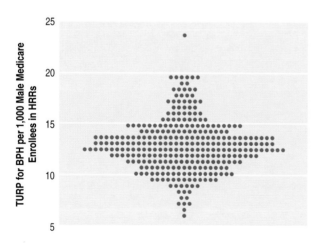

Among hospital referral regions with low rates of TURP per thousand male Medicare enrollees were Augusta, Georgia (6.5); Grand Junction, Colorado (7.1); St. Joseph, Michigan (7.3); Anchorage, Alaska (7.3); Reno, Nevada (7.5); San Francisco (9.2); and New Haven, Connecticut (9.4).

Figure 6.9. TURP for BPH Among Hospital Referral Regions (1992-93)

The rate of TURP varied from fewer than 6 per thousand male Medicare enrollees to more than 23, after adjustment for differences in population age and race. Each point represents one of the 306 hospital referral regions in the United States.

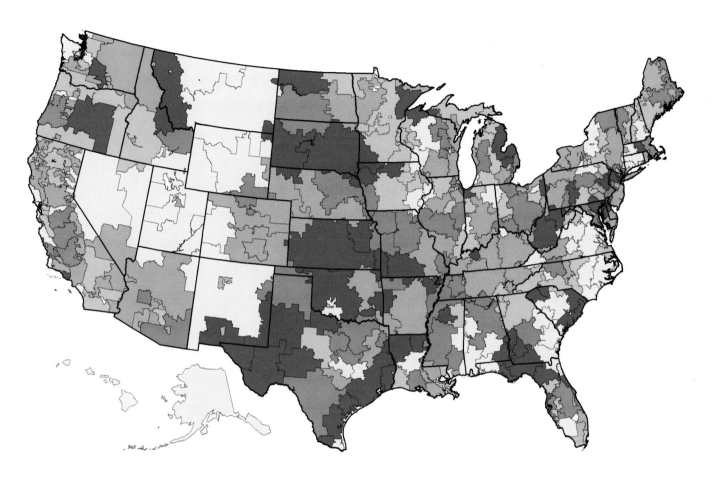

Map 6.9. Transurethral Resection of the Prostate

The rates of TURP among male Medicare enrollees were higher in the Midwest than in most of the rest of the United States, although some areas in the Northwest and Southeast also had high rates. The rates were not uniform among major metropolitan areas: San Francisco had low rates for the procedure, while New York, Washington, and Chicago had high rates.

Transurethral Prostatectomies for Benign Prostatic Hyperplasia per 1,000 Male Medicare Enrollees

by Hospital Referral Region (1992-93)

- 14.62 to 23.70 (61 HRRs)
- 13.31 to <14.62 (61)
- 12.24 to <13.31 (61)
- 10.86 to <12.24 (61)
- 5.84 to <10.86 (62)
- Not Populated

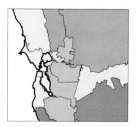

San Francisco

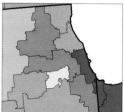

Chicago

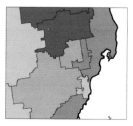

Detroit

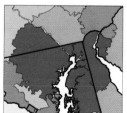

Washington-Baltimore

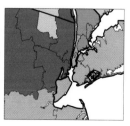

New York

PART SEVEN

Benchmarking

Benchmarking

For years, health policy experts, educators, and professional societies have struggled with the question of how many physicians, nurses, and other health care resources such as hospital beds are "needed." The issue of need has sometimes been framed in terms of the outcomes of care: How much is needed to maximize the health of the American people? Sometimes the issue of need has been placed in the context of demand: How much health care do the American people want?

In recent years, the concept of needs-based or demand-based planning has come under serious challenge, in part because the problem of scientific uncertainty about the outcomes of care has been more widely recognized. The detailed knowledge required to calculate the resources necessary to optimize health status is simply not available. It is also not clear how much care Americans really want. The evidence that provider, rather than patient, preferences dominate much of clinical decision making, and that capacity exercises a threshold effect on utilization, raises serious doubts about the belief that utilization rates reflect patient demand.

In the absence of a detailed understanding of the nature of health care needs, medical care outcomes, and what patients want, what guidelines are available for use in establishing appropriate levels of supply? One method is to examine the way resources are actually used, and to use as "benchmarks" efficiently operated health care plans or communities that appear to have an adequate but not excessive level of supply.

Benchmarking provides answers to two related questions: How much more (or less) health care capacity would the nation need, if all regions had the level of capacity of the benchmark region or health plan? And how much more (or less) health care capacity would be required in a specific region if its per capita capacity were equal to the level of the benchmark region or health plan?

Two useful benchmarks are the Minneapolis hospital referral region and a large, well-established, and successful health maintenance organization. Both have demonstrated the ability to deliver an adequate level of care for defined populations within reasonable constraints. Benchmarking involves the search for communities and health plans that exhibit models of "best practice" – exemplary ways of practicing medicine that provide answers to the question "Which rate is right?"

For a number of common conditions, patient preference is the key to rational choice among alternative treatments, including surgery. The search for "best practices" to benchmark the rates of surgery leads to those practices that have adopted shared decision making, because learning which rate is right requires the active participation of the patient in the decision process. The experiences of two large health maintenance organizations that adopted shared decision making provide a benchmark for the demand for surgical management of benign prostatic hyperplasia (BPH) when patients were empowered to choose among available treatments according to their own preferences.

Benchmarking the United States Supply of Physicians to a Large Health Maintenance Organization

How many physicians would the nation need if supply were geared to meet the requirements of a large staff model health maintenance organization? The supply of physicians in such health maintenance organizations is determined by a deliberate planning process that pays close attention to the ratios of physicians to members. The success of health maintenance organizations in gaining market share has demonstrated that these physician staffing ratios are acceptable to large numbers of consumers.

The impact of using this standard in determining the nation's need for physicians could be substantial; after adjustment for differences in population age, sex, and race, the number of clinically active physicians in the United States in 1993 exceeded by 158,866, or 51%, the number who would have been employed under the physician-to-population hiring ratios used by one large staff model health maintenance organization with more than 2.4 million enrollees.

According to this standard, even the supply of primary care physicians practicing in the United States exceeds the numbers required by the health maintenance organization by 24,403, or 17%. The number of specialists is substantially in excess: 131,065 physicians, or 76%.

The impact would be greater on some specialties than on others. Among the specialties included in Figure 7.1, the per capita number of cardiologists and general surgeons exceeded the number "needed" by more than 100%; by this benchmark, the national supply in 1993 exceeded the health maintenance organization "demand" by more than 8,000 cardiologists and 12,800 general surgeons. The national supply of orthopedic surgeons exceeded the benchmark by 60%; obstetrician/gynecologists by 38%; ophthalmologists by 31%; anesthesiologists by 26%; and urologists by 18%. Radiology was the only one of the listed specialty areas in which the national per capita supply approximated the staffing levels in the health maintenance organization.

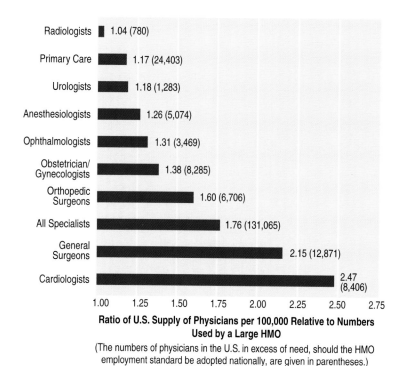

Radiologists ▮ 1.04 (780)
Primary Care 1.17 (24,403)
Urologists 1.18 (1,283)
Anesthesiologists 1.26 (5,074)
Ophthalmologists 1.31 (3,469)
Obstetrician/ Gynecologists 1.38 (8,285)
Orthopedic Surgeons 1.60 (6,706)
All Specialists 1.76 (131,065)
General Surgeons 2.15 (12,871)
Cardiologists 2.47 (8,406)

1.00   1.25   1.50   1.75   2.00   2.25   2.50   2.75

Ratio of U.S. Supply of Physicians per 100,000 Relative to Numbers Used by a Large HMO

(The numbers of physicians in the U.S. in excess of need, should the HMO employment standard be adopted nationally, are given in parentheses.)

Figure 7.1. Ratios of the Rates of Supply of Physicians in the United States to Rates in a Large Health Maintenance Organization (1993)

The supply of physicians per capita for selected specialties in the United States (the numerator) is compared to the number employed by a large staff model health maintenance organization (the denominator). The rates for the health maintenance organization were age and sex adjusted to take into account differences between the United States population and the population served by the health maintenance organization. For example, the national supply of cardiologists per hundred thousand population exceeds the number employed by the health maintenance organization by 147%. The numbers in parentheses indicate the excess number of physicians in the United States workforce, according to the health maintenance organization benchmark. According to this benchmark, there are 8,406 more cardiologists practicing in the United States than are required to meet the needs of staff model health maintenance organizations.

Benchmarking the United States Supply of Physicians to the Minneapolis Hospital Referral Region

Another way of looking at "need" is to examine how many physicians are in active practice in selected hospital referral regions, and to use those regions as benchmarks. This approach has the advantage of measuring the workforce that is providing care to everyone living in the region, including people with special needs (such as those with chronic illnesses) who are not eligible for health maintenance organization membership, and those who are institutionalized in mental hospitals. The estimate for need varies substantially, depending on the region selected as the benchmark. For example, the per capita physician workforce serving San Francisco in 1993 was 68% above the national average. If the levels of staffing in San Francisco were the standard for the nation, an additional 318,800 physicians would be needed. By contrast, the per capita physician workforce serving Dayton, Ohio, was only 78% of the national average. If Dayton's supply were the standard for the United States, the nation would have an excess of 103,500 physicians.

We have used the Minneapolis hospital referral region, which has a strong penetration of managed care, as the regional benchmark for this Atlas. According to the Minneapolis benchmark, the national per capita supply of primary care physicians in 1993 was not sufficient to meet existing needs. The national rate of primary care physicians per hundred thousand population was 93% of the staffing level in Minneapolis; to raise the primary physician-to-population ratio of the nation as a whole to the same level, 12,056 additional primary care physicians would be needed.

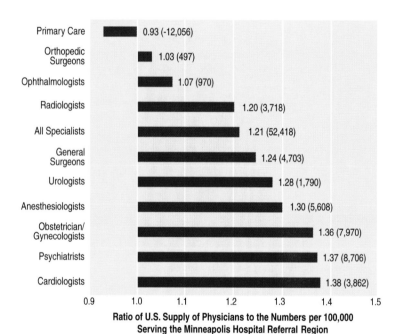

Ratio of U.S. Supply of Physicians to the Numbers per 100,000
Serving the Minneapolis Hospital Referral Region

(The numbers of physicians in the U.S. in excess (+) or deficit (-) of need, should the
Minneapolis benchmark be adopted nationally, are given in parentheses.)

Figure 7.2. Ratios of the Rates of Supply of Physicians in the United States to Rates in the Minneapolis Hospital Referral Region (1993)

The per capita physician workforce in Minneapolis was lower than the national level of supply in every specialty. If the Minneapolis benchmark were the standard for the nation, the per capita supply of cardiologists would exceed need by 38%, and there would be an excess of 3,862 cardiologists in the United States workforce.

The national supply of specialists in 1993 exceeded the staffing pattern in Minneapolis by 21%, or 52,418 specialists. Among the individual specialties listed in Figure 7.2, the national per capita supplies for obstetrician/gynecologists, cardiologists, anesthesiologists, and psychiatrists exceeded the numbers required to achieve the Minneapolis benchmark by at least 30%; the supplies of general surgeons, radiologists, and urologists were 20% to 28% higher than the Minneapolis benchmark. Orthopedic surgery was the only listed specialty in which the national per capita supply approximated the numbers used by the residents of the Minneapolis hospital referral region.

There were important differences between the staff model health maintenance organization and the Minneapolis region in the per capita supply and composition of the physician workforce. The number of primary care physicians serving Minneapolis exceeded the health maintenance organization benchmark by 26% (Figure 7.3). Although the number of all specialists available in the Minneapolis hospital referral region exceeded the health maintenance organization benchmark by 46%, the health maintenance organization had a greater supply of some specialists, including radiologists (16%), urologists (8%), and anesthesiologists (3%). By contrast, the per capita number of cardiologists exceeded the health maintenance organization benchmark by 79%, and the number of general surgeons by 73%.

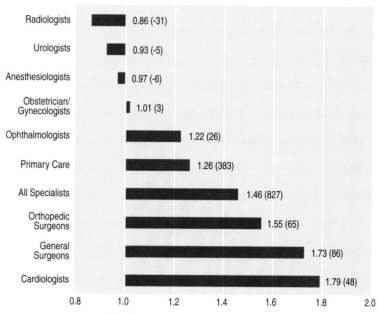

Ratio of Minneapolis Supply of Physicians to the Numbers per 100,000 Used by a Large HMO

(The numbers of physicians in the Minneapolis HRR in excess (+) or deficit (-) of need, should the HMO benchmark be adopted for Minneapolis, are given in parentheses.)

Figure 7.3. Ratios of the Rates of Supply of Physicians in Minneapolis to Rates in a Large Health Maintenance Organization (1993)

The rates were age and sex adjusted to take into account differences in age structure.

The number of primary care physicians serving the Minneapolis region exceeded the health maintenance organization benchmark by 26%. The numbers in parentheses are the numbers of physicians working in the Minneapolis region in excess of (+) or below (-) the health maintenance organization standard. (For example, if Minneapolis were to have the same per capita supply of primary care physicians as the health maintenance organization, it would need to reduce its primary care workforce by 383 physicians.) The Minneapolis region had fewer physicians per hundred thousand population practicing in some specialties than the health maintenance organization; for example, according to the health maintenance organization benchmark, Minneapolis had a shortage of 31 radiologists.

Benchmarking Medicare Reimbursements and the Supply of Hospital Resources in the United States to the Minneapolis Hospital Referral Region

Benchmarking can be applied to Medicare reimbursements as well as to the supply of acute care hospital resources and physicians. In 1993, Medicare program outlays were more than $115 billion for beneficiaries 65 years of age and older served by fee-for-service providers. The national per enrollee reimbursement rate exceeded the rate for the Minneapolis hospital referral region by 40% (Figure 7.4). The price adjusted Minneapolis rate was well below the United States average for each sector of care. Overall, if the spending experience for Minneapolis had been the standard for the nation, federal reimbursements would have been $32.6 billion lower. The greatest savings would have been for professional and laboratory services ($14.7 billion), followed by inpatient hospital services ($10.2 billion), home health care services ($6.1 billion), and outpatient services ($1.0 billion).

The supplies of acute care hospital beds, full time equivalent employees, and hospital-based registered nurses in the Minneapolis hospital referral region were also substantially below the United States average in 1993. In that year, there were more than 825,000 staffed acute care hospital beds allocated to the populations living in the 306 hospital referral regions in the United States. If the Minneapolis benchmark for use of acute care hospital beds had been the standard for the nation, national capacity could have been reduced by almost 120,000 beds, or 14.5%. In the same year, the nation's hospitals employed more than 3,555,000 full time equivalent workers; if the Minneapolis employment levels had been the benchmark for the nation, the workforce could have been reduced by about 768,000, or 21.9%. Acute care hospitals in the United States employed more than 872,000 registered nurses in 1993; if the Minneapolis nurse staffing level had applied to the entire United States in that year, the excess supply of nurses would have been more than 187,000, or 21.4%.

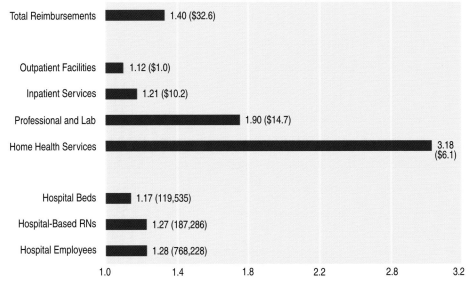

Ratio of U.S. Supply of Hospital Resources and Expenditures and
Medicare Reimbursements to Minneapolis HRR Benchmarks

(The amounts of resources, and billions of dollars in expenditures and reimbursements
in excess of the Minneapolis benchmarks are given in parentheses.)

**Figure 7.4. Ratios of the Rates for Medicare Reimbursements and for Hospital Resource Allocations
in the United States to the Rates in the Minneapolis Hospital Referral Region (1993)**
*There would be substantial savings in both Medicare reimbursements and hospital resources if the experience in the
Minneapolis hospital referral region were the standard for the nation. Rates of resource allocation and
reimbursements have been age, sex, and race adjusted. The numbers in parentheses are the savings in billions of
dollars or the resources (beds and personnel) in excess of need if the Minneapolis experience were the standard for
the nation.*

Benchmarking the Chicago, Los Angeles, New Orleans, Miami, and Philadelphia
Hospital Referral Regions to the Minneapolis Hospital Referral Region

The information presented in this Atlas makes it possible to answer very specific
questions about resource allocation. By how much does the supply of hospital resources serving one region differ from another region? How many more (or fewer)
physicians would be required if the practice patterns in one region were applied to
another?

The per capita number of physicians allocated to the Minneapolis hospital referral region in 1993 was considerably smaller than the numbers allocated to the other regions (Figure 7.5). Philadelphia had 50% more physicians per capita than Minneapolis, and Chicago exceeded the benchmark by 32%. The supply of physicians was 30% higher in New Orleans, 21% higher in Los Angeles, and 38% higher in Miami than in Minneapolis. The per capita numbers of primary care physicians were greater than in Minneapolis in Philadelphia (26%), Chicago (21%), and Miami (17%). By contrast, the rate in New Orleans was only 86 % of that in Minneapolis. The supply of specialists in each region exceeded the benchmark, ranging from 35% in excess in Los Angeles to 68% in Philadelphia. The physician workforce in the Philadelphia region exceeded the numbers that would be employed under the Minneapolis model for resource allocation by more than 3,400. In contrast, New Orleans would have needed 82 more primary care physicians to reach the Minneapolis benchmark.

Acute care hospital services and Medicare reimbursements exceeded the Minneapolis benchmark in each of the five regions (Figure 7.6). Age, sex, race and price adjusted Medi

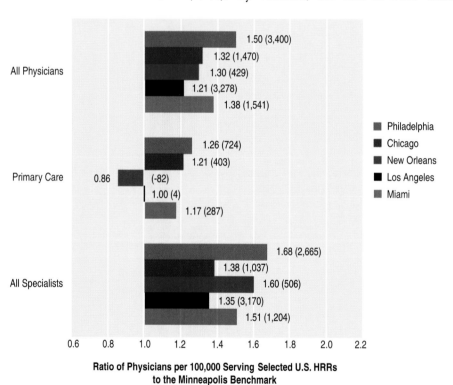

Ratio of Physicians per 100,000 Serving Selected U.S. HRRs to the Minneapolis Benchmark

(The numbers of physicians serving each selected HRR in excess (+) or in deficit (-) of need, should the Minneapolis benchmark be adopted, are given in parentheses.)

Figure 7.5. Ratios of the Rates of Physicians in Selected HRRs to Rates in the Minneapolis Hospital Referral Region (1993)

The supply of all physicians per hundred thousand residents in Philadelphia exceeded the supply in Minneapolis by 50%. Rates were age and sex adjusted. If Philadelphia's rate were to be reduced to the rate in Minneapolis, 3,400 fewer physicians would be needed. The numbers in parentheses are the numbers of physicians working in the selected cities in excess of (+) or below (-) the Minneapolis benchmark.

care reimbursements in the Miami region exceeded those in the Minneapolis region by 130%. If reimbursements in Miami in 1993 had been at the per capita rate of the Minneapolis region, federal outlays for care in Miami would have been $860 million less. The per capita numbers of hospital beds and hospital employees in the Chicago region exceeded those for Minneapolis by 61% and 88%, respectively. If Chicago had had the bed supply and hospital employee ratios of Minneapolis, the region would have used 4,625 fewer beds and 26,338 fewer hospital employees.

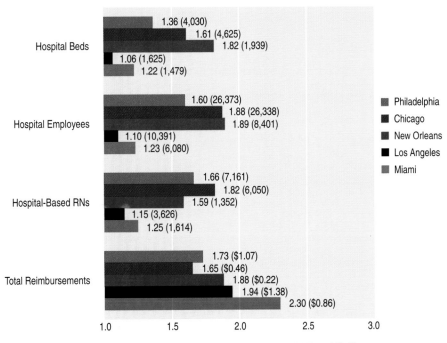

Ratio of Quantities of Hospital Resources per 1,000 and Medicare Reimbursements per capita in Selected U.S. HRRs to the Minneapolis Benchmark

(The amounts of hospital resources and billions of Medicare dollars that would be saved in each selected HRR, should the Minneapolis benchmark be adopted, are given in parentheses.)

Figure 7.6. Ratios of the Rates for Hospital Resources and Medicare Reimbursement in Selected HRRs to Rates in the Minneapolis Hospital Referral Region (1993).

Resource allocations greatly exceeded the level in Minneapolis. The acute care hospital bed capacity per thousand residents in New Orleans exceeded the supply in Minneapolis by 82%. If New Orleans' rate for beds per thousand residents had been reduced to the rate in Minneapolis, 1,939 beds could have been eliminated. The numbers in parentheses are the amount of hospital resources or of Medicare reimbursements that would have been saved if the referenced region had been equal to the Minneapolis benchmark. (Medicare reimbursements are for Medicare beneficiaries served by fee-for-service providers, including non-risk bearing health maintenance organizations.) Rates were age, sex, and race adjusted.

Benchmarking the Rates of Surgery

Learning which rate of surgery is right depends on making fundamental changes in the provider-patient relationship. Patients must participate as active partners in decision making, and health plans must deal with the problem of unwanted provider influence on demand. The experiences of two staff model health maintenance organizations that adopted shared decision making for benign prostatic hyperplasia (BPH) provide a benchmark for estimating the demand for prostatectomy. After adopting shared decision making, the plans' rates of transurethral prostatectomy (TURP) dropped about 40%, even though their rates were already well below the national average. If the preferences of men throughout the United States proved similar to those of men enrolled in the two health maintenance organizations, the demand for the procedure under shared decision making would be substantially less than the amount delivered under traditional Medicare in 1992-93. In 1992-93, only the Augusta, Georgia, and Bryan, Texas, hospital referral regions had rates of TURP that were within 10% of the health maintenance organizations' benchmark.

These benchmarks do not take into account the longer-range experience under shared decision making and therefore might underestimate the "steady state" surgery rate, since patients can change their minds and choose surgery after the initial period of watchful waiting. On the other hand, the rates reflect demand in practice settings where no extra fee was paid when patients chose surgical care; the health maintenance organizations' experience therefore overestimates demand in situations where patients are asked to share the costs of surgery.

The importance of benchmarking the rates of use of surgery under shared decision making is illustrated in Figure 7.7. The figure includes nine conditions for which the rates of surgery vary substantially from region to region. Surgical treatment of these conditions accounts for more than half of the costs of surgery performed in the United States.

Figure 7.7. Conditions for Which Patient Preferences Are Important for Rational Choice Among Treatment Options

Conditions	Major Treatment Options
Angina pectoris	Bypass surgery vs. angioplasty vs. drugs
Arthritis of hip and knee	Hip/knee replacement vs. medical management
Atherosclerosis of carotid artery with threat of stroke	Carotid endarterectomy vs. aspirin
Benign prostatic hyperplasia (BPH)	Surgery (by type) vs. drugs vs. microwave diathermy vs. watchful waiting
Cataracts	Lens extraction (by type) vs. watchful waiting
Gallstones	Surgery vs. stone crushing vs. medical management vs. watchful waiting
Herniated disc	Surgery (by type) vs. various medical management strategies
Peripheral vascular disease	Bypass surgery vs. angioplasty vs. medical management
Symptoms of menopause	Surgery (by type) vs. hormone treatments vs. drugs vs. watchful waiting

Part Eight

Tables

The tables in this part of the Atlas provide specific information for each hospital referral region. Most, but not all, of the data displayed in maps and figures in parts One through Seven are presented here. Tables One and Two provide estimates of acute care hospital resources and the physician workforce allocated to hospital referral regions. In these tables, the rates are for the resident population of the regions. In tables Three and Four, the rates are for Medicare enrollees who are not members of risk bearing health maintenance organizations. Table Three provides rates for hospitalizations, diagnostic and surgical procedures, and mortality. Table Four contains reimbursement rates for the various components of the Medicare program.

The tables provide the information necessary for benchmarking any hospital referral region to another or to the national average. Readers interested in benchmarking are referred to Part Nine, Section 3.9, which contains instructions on how to do the calculations for any given region.

For readability, the data in the tables have been rounded, usually to one place to the right of the decimal point.

Description of Variables for Table 1

Variable	Description	Price Adjustment	Figure List
Total Population	Based on 1990 Census. All ages.		
Adjusted Beds per 1000	Allocated and Age, Sex, Adjusted Beds per 1000 of Total Population		2.1, 3.1, 3.3, 3.4, 3.5, 3.6, 3.7, 3.8, 7.4, 7.6
Adjusted FTE per 1000	Allocated and Age, Sex, Adjusted Full Time Equivalent Hospital Employees per 1000 of Total Population		2.2, 3.2, 7.4, 7.6
Adjusted RNs per 1000	Allocated and Age, Sex, Adjusted Registered Nurses per 1000 of Total Population		2.3, 7.4, 7.6
Adjusted Total Expenditures per Capita	Price Adjusted, Allocated, and Age, Sex Adjusted Total Hospital Expenditures per Capita for the Total Population	Price Index for total population	2.4, 3.1

Acute Care Hospital Resources Allocated to Hospital Referral Regions

(Rates for 1993)*

Hospital Referral Region	Resident Population	Acute Care Beds per 1000	Hospital Employees per 1000	Hospital-based Registered Nurses per 1000	Expenditures per capita
Alabama					
Birmingham	1,983,947	4.3	16.3	4.0	1,228
Dothan	328,197	4.3	14.2	3.3	1,170
Huntsville	472,826	3.7	13.6	3.6	970
Mobile	680,935	4.3	16.2	4.1	1,223
Montgomery	398,081	3.6	13.7	3.5	985
Tuscaloosa	228,294	3.8	16.4	3.6	1,169
Alaska					
Anchorage	546,182	3.8	17.3	4.8	1,232
Arizona					
Mesa	683,368	1.9	8.0	2.4	670
Phoenix	1,937,465	2.8	12.4	3.1	1,005
Sun City	133,419	2.8	9.3	2.3	780
Tucson	838,882	2.4	10.8	2.6	856
Arkansas					
Fort Smith	303,027	3.9	12.5	2.8	877
Jonesboro	200,076	3.4	11.9	2.8	953
Little Rock	1,321,705	4.1	15.2	3.7	1,148
Springdale	295,913	2.9	13.7	3.0	862
Texarkana	245,516	4.5	14.9	3.4	1,215
California					
Orange Co.	2,561,917	2.6	10.1	2.9	808
Bakersfield	753,777	2.5	12.3	3.0	984
Chico	247,777	2.3	12.9	3.6	1,032
Contra Costa Co.	776,882	2.1	9.7	2.7	837
Fresno	870,093	2.3	12.2	2.7	960
Los Angeles	8,891,233	3.0	12.4	3.2	970
Modesto	642,363	2.8	11.7	3.0	1,015
Napa	237,369	2.8	13.6	3.0	1,064
Alameda Co.	1,307,511	2.3	10.5	2.8	898
Palm Spr/Rancho Mir	214,236	2.6	12.1	2.5	1,114
Redding	291,627	2.7	12.2	3.9	1,098
Sacramento	1,826,537	2.1	10.7	2.9	866
Salinas	340,435	2.1	10.4	2.4	1,024
San Bernardino	2,052,460	2.6	11.3	3.1	891
San Diego	2,767,527	2.1	9.8	2.5	764
San Francisco	1,281,325	2.6	12.9	3.1	1,038
San Jose	1,463,526	2.1	9.3	2.7	788
San Luis Obispo	205,889	2.5	9.6	2.8	711
San Mateo Co.	723,533	2.0	10.0	2.5	791
Santa Barbara	374,609	2.3	8.6	2.3	665
Santa Cruz	240,944	1.9	7.2	2.0	667
Santa Rosa	393,669	2.0	8.4	2.4	714
Stockton	413,152	2.6	12.7	3.4	1,007
Ventura	700,513	2.1	10.0	2.6	700
Colorado					
Boulder	212,469	2.1	12.1	3.2	818
Colorado Springs	561,723	3.0	13.3	3.2	929
Denver	1,904,201	3.0	13.4	3.5	1,018
Fort Collins	238,089	2.6	10.5	2.5	838
Grand Junction	201,585	2.6	12.1	3.3	973
Greeley	227,007	2.9	13.9	3.7	1,062
Pueblo	133,475	3.0	12.6	2.8	875
Connecticut					
Bridgeport	629,535	2.7	12.5	2.8	837
Hartford	1,393,087	2.7	13.5	3.2	916
New Haven	1,349,858	2.5	12.6	2.8	851
Delaware					
Wilmington	635,637	3.1	16.4	4.2	1,166
District of Columbia					
Washington	2,153,979	3.3	15.5	4.0	1,063
Florida					
Bradenton	197,705	2.9	7.9	1.9	698
Clearwater	450,255	2.8	8.9	2.3	749
Fort Lauderdale	1,927,706	3.0	11.2	2.9	893
Fort Myers	627,321	3.0	11.8	2.8	997
Gainesville	407,508	3.1	12.3	2.9	1,007
Hudson	287,224	3.0	9.9	2.3	846
Jacksonville	1,137,244	3.5	15.1	3.8	1,159
Lakeland	279,997	2.3	10.3	2.6	853
Miami	2,365,502	3.5	13.8	3.4	993
Ocala	292,949	2.5	10.5	2.6	880
Orlando	2,251,255	3.0	12.8	3.0	952
Ormond Beach	268,338	2.9	11.1	2.7	875
Panama City	161,325	3.4	14.6	3.3	1,069
Pensacola	588,018	4.1	13.5	3.3	1,026
Sarasota	317,728	2.6	10.1	2.2	848
St Petersburg	401,404	3.5	12.6	3.2	918

Hospital Referral Region	Resident Population	Acute Care Beds per 1000	Hospital Employees per 1000	Hospital-based Registered Nurses per 1000	Expenditures per capita
Tallahassee	628,832	3.8	14.4	2.9	990
Tampa	876,408	3.1	11.9	3.2	967
Georgia					
Albany	200,455	4.1	14.9	3.0	1,063
Atlanta	3,700,835	3.4	14.9	3.8	1,112
Augusta	548,493	4.2	17.3	3.8	1,278
Columbus	301,665	4.9	13.7	2.7	1,060
Macon	597,635	4.1	16.5	3.4	1,211
Rome	220,157	3.6	13.6	3.4	1,015
Savannah	601,416	3.9	16.7	3.3	1,253
Hawaii					
Honolulu	1,108,229	2.4	13.6	3.1	992
Idaho					
Boise	517,555	2.6	12.4	3.4	896
Idaho Falls	166,131	3.1	12.3	3.4	930
Illinois					
Aurora	181,602	2.7	9.8	2.6	719
Blue Island	805,400	3.5	15.5	3.7	1,164
Chicago	2,680,712	4.6	21.0	5.0	1,475
Elgin	522,152	2.6	11.3	3.0	874
Evanston	861,134	2.8	14.1	3.8	991
Hinsdale	341,601	2.5	12.1	3.4	932
Joliet	438,832	3.8	15.8	3.6	1,107
Melrose Park	1,189,327	3.0	14.2	3.7	1,077
Peoria	601,129	3.5	16.1	3.8	1,208
Rockford	623,702	3.2	13.7	3.7	1,004
Springfield	820,868	3.8	15.6	3.4	1,095
Urbana	429,114	3.0	12.9	3.3	995
Bloomington	163,421	2.6	13.8	3.0	1,138
Indiana					
Evansville	646,627	4.0	15.3	3.9	1,061
Fort Wayne	767,226	3.2	13.2	3.3	978
Gary	485,735	4.5	17.1	3.6	1,319
Indianapolis	2,324,142	3.5	17.0	4.1	1,220
Lafayette	197,673	2.8	13.7	3.4	977
Muncie	171,507	3.3	12.6	2.6	1,034
Munster	296,292	4.6	19.1	4.7	1,476
South Bend	611,180	2.9	12.6	3.6	992
Terre Haute	176,806	3.6	15.0	4.0	1,077
Iowa					
Cedar Rapids	252,695	3.9	14.9	4.7	1,011
Davenport	486,583	3.9	14.0	3.8	1,072
Des Moines	928,747	3.9	15.1	3.5	1,121
Dubuque	147,879	3.4	14.0	3.9	937
Iowa City	308,514	3.5	15.3	4.2	1,122
Mason City	143,369	2.1	6.5	1.6	503
Sioux City	252,103	3.8	13.9	3.6	1,055

Hospital Referral Region	Resident Population	Acute Care Beds per 1000	Hospital Employees per 1000	Hospital-based Registered Nurses per 1000	Expenditures per capita
Waterloo	205,443	3.6	14.6	3.6	1,043
Kansas					
Topeka	421,682	3.2	11.9	3.3	826
Wichita	1,169,518	4.1	14.6	3.6	1,051
Kentucky					
Covington	316,933	3.3	14.7	4.0	975
Lexington	1,290,244	3.9	14.4	3.6	1,071
Louisville	1,464,748	3.8	14.5	3.8	1,104
Owensboro	131,949	4.2	15.9	3.7	1,143
Paducah	342,954	4.3	16.8	3.9	1,206
Louisiana					
Alexandria	277,018	4.4	17.2	3.7	1,256
Baton Rouge	734,846	3.8	14.8	3.5	1,110
Houma	245,201	4.1	16.2	3.0	1,220
Lafayette	535,796	4.6	16.5	3.1	1,172
Lake Charles	258,157	4.6	17.3	3.5	1,261
Metairie	396,726	4.6	18.3	4.1	1,404
Monroe	266,139	5.3	24.0	4.4	1,356
New Orleans	838,284	5.2	21.2	4.4	1,646
Shreveport	646,435	4.3	15.5	3.1	1,228
Slidell	140,609	4.3	15.8	3.7	1,147
Maine					
Bangor	396,634	3.3	15.5	4.1	1,066
Portland	948,869	2.9	13.2	3.3	939
Maryland					
Baltimore	2,247,761	3.3	16.7	4.2	1,116
Salisbury	305,907	3.2	15.2	3.7	998
Takoma Park	778,169	2.5	10.7	3.1	703
Massachusetts					
Boston	4,418,982	3.1	16.7	3.7	1,202
Springfield	727,784	2.8	13.0	3.1	953
Worcester	711,982	2.7	13.4	3.1	908
Michigan					
Ann Arbor	1,192,620	2.8	14.1	3.2	1,015
Dearborn	524,139	3.5	15.8	3.4	1,085
Detroit	1,937,050	3.7	18.8	4.3	1,263
Flint	550,338	4.0	17.0	3.7	1,226
Grand Rapids	954,534	2.5	12.0	3.3	865
Kalamazoo	620,043	2.8	13.0	3.4	1,022
Lansing	647,965	3.1	15.3	3.5	1,088
Marquette	202,537	3.9	14.2	2.8	1,094
Muskegon	241,421	3.2	12.2	2.8	1,000
Petoskey	148,605	3.3	12.7	3.5	942
Pontiac	391,240	3.1	15.5	3.6	1,082
Royal Oak	650,771	2.7	17.7	4.0	1,105
Saginaw	628,840	3.6	16.3	3.6	1,147
St Joseph	145,896	3.2	16.4	3.7	1,086

Hospital Referral Region	Resident Population	Acute Care Beds per 1000	Hospital Employees per 1000	Hospital-based Registered Nurses per 1000	Expenditures per capita
Traverse City	177,508	3.4	15.7	3.7	1,148
Minnesota					
Duluth	323,298	3.4	12.4	2.8	988
Minneapolis	2,614,660	2.8	11.2	2.8	916
Rochester	363,251	3.2	10.4	3.1	796
St Cloud	205,700	3.0	11.6	2.5	915
St Paul	840,098	2.8	11.0	2.9	982
Mississippi					
Gulfport	175,723	4.5	15.5	4.7	1,190
Hattiesburg	252,292	4.8	17.2	4.0	1,190
Jackson	979,993	4.7	15.3	3.2	989
Meridian	192,396	5.0	18.4	4.3	1,252
Oxford	129,317	4.9	17.0	3.2	1,138
Tupelo	349,277	4.4	15.5	3.5	1,086
Missouri					
Cape Girardeau	253,402	3.4	14.5	3.4	1,038
Columbia	587,088	3.7	15.9	3.6	1,230
Joplin	311,296	4.0	15.5	3.8	1,139
Kansas City	2,025,703	3.3	14.6	3.7	1,072
Springfield	619,065	3.4	14.5	3.7	1,010
St Louis	3,134,871	4.0	17.4	4.1	1,246
Montana					
Billings	463,221	3.4	13.6	3.2	1,050
Great Falls	148,937	4.3	18.2	3.6	1,292
Missoula	288,550	3.1	13.1	3.2	1,042
Nebraska					
Lincoln	508,894	3.6	12.2	2.8	909
Omaha	1,119,894	3.8	15.2	3.6	1,172
Nevada					
Las Vegas	794,033	3.1	10.3	2.9	907
Reno	483,100	3.0	13.2	3.3	1,079
New Hampshire					
Lebanon	363,701	3.3	14.4	3.7	1,282
Manchester	740,593	2.5	11.7	3.1	900
New Jersey					
Camden	2,454,954	3.5	15.0	3.8	1,018
Hackensack	1,129,751	3.7	14.7	3.8	912
Morristown	878,642	3.1	12.6	2.8	816
New Brunswick	838,495	3.2	13.9	3.3	849
Newark	1,466,813	4.7	19.0	4.4	1,241
Paterson	364,246	3.6	15.3	3.6	946
Ridgewood	379,311	2.9	12.0	3.3	752
New Mexico					
Albuquerque	1,254,781	3.1	15.5	3.9	1,205
New York					
Albany	1,721,696	3.4	13.9	3.3	893
Binghamton	376,954	2.9	13.4	3.0	911
Bronx	1,211,361	4.9	26.4	5.4	1,682
Buffalo	1,437,600	3.6	16.4	3.8	979
Elmira	344,696	3.3	14.5	3.6	932
East Long Island	4,242,448	3.3	14.7	3.6	936
New York	4,568,777	4.6	22.3	4.8	1,467
Rochester	1,243,904	3.1	15.4	3.4	914
Syracuse	1,074,023	3.1	13.7	3.2	882
White Plains	1,025,646	3.5	13.9	3.8	884
North Carolina					
Asheville	490,407	2.9	13.5	3.5	958
Charlotte	1,558,895	3.1	13.8	3.6	989
Durham	1,044,489	3.2	16.2	3.2	1,169
Greensboro	473,708	2.9	13.4	3.8	912
Greenville	696,239	3.3	14.0	3.7	1,024
Hickory	236,085	3.3	14.3	4.1	1,056
Raleigh	1,279,158	3.0	13.2	3.3	966
Wilmington	277,569	3.5	16.2	3.9	1,129
Winston-Salem	883,657	3.3	14.4	3.8	985
North Dakota					
Bismarck	201,983	5.2	17.0	4.5	1,318
Fargo Moorhead -Mn	464,935	3.4	12.4	3.3	975
Grand Forks	179,647	4.1	15.8	3.5	1,099
Minot	127,785	4.9	16.0	3.5	1,236
Ohio					
Akron	668,249	3.4	16.4	4.4	1,280
Canton	602,501	3.3	12.7	3.2	975
Cincinnati	1,509,444	3.4	16.3	4.1	1,278
Cleveland	2,086,998	3.6	16.0	3.9	1,155
Columbus	2,525,830	3.2	14.7	3.7	1,146
Dayton	1,111,678	3.6	15.9	4.2	1,123
Elyria	241,159	3.7	14.4	3.7	978
Kettering	360,768	3.1	13.4	3.6	961
Toledo	982,485	3.7	17.4	4.7	1,317
Youngstown	688,740	4.0	16.8	4.3	1,325
Oklahoma					
Lawton	192,373	3.5	13.4	2.3	974
Oklahoma City	1,565,094	3.8	14.8	3.2	1,031
Tulsa	1,140,749	3.6	14.4	3.1	964
Oregon					
Bend	121,666	2.9	11.9	4.2	954
Eugene	604,042	2.2	10.6	3.1	875
Medford	338,364	2.4	11.3	2.6	857
Portland	1,894,661	2.2	10.5	3.2	856
Salem	227,361	2.0	10.1	3.1	727
Pennsylvania					
Allentown	985,564	3.2	13.7	3.8	918
Altoona	297,507	3.1	13.9	3.4	1,066

Hospital Referral Region	Resident Population	Acute Care Beds per 1000	Hospital Employees per 1000	Hospital-based Registered Nurses per 1000	Expenditures per capita
Danville	536,017	3.5	14.3	3.5	1,053
Erie	732,505	4.0	14.4	3.7	1,065
Harrisburg	879,941	2.8	12.8	3.2	939
Johnstown	241,968	3.8	19.0	4.9	1,411
Lancaster	529,921	2.6	12.1	2.9	817
Philadelphia	3,921,220	3.9	17.9	4.6	1,295
Pittsburgh	3,055,252	4.0	17.5	4.5	1,315
Reading	510,057	2.9	12.6	3.1	859
Sayre	191,385	3.4	13.3	3.6	899
Scranton	300,457	3.3	13.9	3.6	1,025
Wilkes-Barre	258,306	3.7	13.7	3.5	975
York	340,946	2.4	12.6	2.9	879
Rhode Island					
Providence	1,151,761	2.8	13.5	3.1	896
South Carolina					
Charleston	742,214	3.6	15.5	4.0	1,303
Columbia	980,780	3.2	14.4	3.8	1,077
Florence	333,436	3.9	16.8	3.8	1,326
Greenville	682,364	2.7	11.9	2.8	1,038
Spartanburg	306,233	3.8	14.8	3.5	1,100
South Dakota					
Rapid City	184,008	4.1	16.4	3.5	1,231
Sioux Falls	699,852	4.2	13.7	3.7	1,079
Tennessee					
Chattanooga	563,958	3.5	15.6	4.3	1,231
Jackson	287,699	4.0	13.9	3.3	1,038
Johnson City	217,622	4.0	13.8	3.5	1,127
Kingsport	464,124	4.2	15.7	3.5	1,250
Knoxville	1,067,260	3.8	16.0	3.5	1,225
Memphis	1,597,501	4.2	16.5	3.6	1,247
Nashville	1,944,017	4.1	15.1	3.7	1,230
Texas					
Abilene	278,103	3.4	13.5	3.1	975
Amarillo	386,240	4.1	15.2	3.7	1,128
Austin	870,567	2.3	9.0	2.3	750
Beaumont	425,872	4.7	17.6	3.7	1,299
Bryan	184,248	2.4	9.8	2.1	903
Corpus Christi	492,319	3.7	15.4	3.0	1,076
Dallas	3,070,082	3.3	13.7	3.6	1,047
El Paso	811,036	2.9	12.0	2.9	1,034
Fort Worth	1,429,666	3.0	13.0	3.4	1,070
Harlingen	377,065	3.2	12.5	2.5	1,037
Houston	4,195,450	4.2	17.3	4.2	1,354
Longview	182,480	2.8	12.5	3.5	930
Lubbock	634,031	4.8	15.8	3.4	1,293
McAllen	324,820	2.7	9.3	2.7	843
Odessa	306,783	3.5	13.8	3.6	1,072

Hospital Referral Region	Resident Population	Acute Care Beds per 1000	Hospital Employees per 1000	Hospital-based Registered Nurses per 1000	Expenditures per capita
San Angelo	150,062	4.0	15.3	3.3	1,086
San Antonio	1,795,095	3.0	12.4	2.9	933
Temple	323,119	2.6	11.9	2.4	729
Tyler	425,534	3.4	15.1	3.3	1,180
Victoria	133,472	4.5	15.1	3.1	1,039
Waco	279,913	2.9	10.7	2.3	807
Wichita Falls	194,271	3.7	12.3	2.3	868
Utah					
Ogden	307,965	3.0	13.7	3.4	977
Provo	312,598	2.7	12.6	3.1	1,026
Salt Lake City	1,376,597	2.8	15.7	4.0	1,069
Vermont					
Burlington	593,348	3.2	13.6	3.4	948
Virginia					
Arlington	1,516,813	2.2	9.1	2.5	651
Charlottesville	431,219	3.0	16.3	4.4	1,159
Lynchburg	213,943	2.8	11.9	3.2	833
Newport News	470,475	3.1	12.0	2.7	886
Norfolk	1,124,582	3.1	13.1	3.5	947
Richmond	1,247,486	3.5	14.5	3.8	1,028
Roanoke	655,809	3.7	15.1	3.5	1,105
Winchester	294,525	3.3	14.5	3.6	897
Washington					
Everett	430,246	2.0	9.6	2.7	823
Olympia	264,075	2.6	10.2	2.6	920
Seattle	2,151,656	2.2	11.1	2.9	914
Spokane	1,083,197	3.0	11.2	3.0	915
Tacoma	589,030	2.3	11.6	2.3	911
Yakima	224,261	2.6	11.4	3.3	951
West Virginia					
Charleston	856,149	4.1	15.8	3.7	1,257
Huntington	349,438	4.2	15.0	4.1	1,161
Morgantown	376,117	3.3	15.2	3.7	1,238
Wisconsin					
Appleton	269,657	2.9	11.2	2.7	847
Green Bay	446,098	2.7	11.9	3.1	890
La Crosse	320,536	3.0	11.6	3.1	840
Madison	875,793	2.9	12.8	3.3	992
Marshfield	342,484	3.4	11.0	2.8	922
Milwaukee	2,326,759	3.0	13.6	3.6	1,042
Neenah	201,177	3.2	13.2	3.3	946
Wausau	167,971	3.0	11.8	2.9	895
Wyoming					
Casper	164,307	5.0	16.6	4.6	1127
United States					
US	248,652,605	3.3	14.3	3.5	1,053

*All rates are age and sex adjusted and corrected for out of area use. Expenditures per capita are also price adjusted. Estimates for numbers of hospital employees and hospital-based registered nurses are for full time equivalents. See Part Nine, Section 2 for details on the methods used for estimating populations and adjusting rates, and for other details concerning the rates in this table.

Description of Variables for Table 2

Variable	Description	Price Adjustment	Figure List
Total Population	Based on 1990 Census. All ages.		
All Physicians	All Allocated Federal and non-Federal Physicians per 100,000 persons in HRRs including the Unspecified Physicians but excluding Resident Physicians		5.1, 7.5
Primary Care Physicians	Allocated Federal and non-Federal Physicians with Specialties of Family Practice, Internal Medicine, and Pediatrics per 100,000 persons in HRRs		5.2, 5.b, 7.1, 7.2, 7.3, 7.5
Specialists	All Allocated Federal and non-Federal Physicians except Primare Care and Unspecified Physicians per 100,000 persons in HRRs		5.3, 5.a, 7.1, 7.2, 7.3, 7.5
Anesthesiologists	See Dartmouth grouping of Specialties		5.4, 7.1, 7.2, 7.3
Cardiologists	"		5.5, 7.1, 7.2, 7.3
General Surgeons	"		5.6, 7.1, 7.2, 7.3
Obstetrician / Gynecologists	"		5.7, 7.1, 7.2, 7.3
Ophthalmologists	"		5.8, 7.1, 7.2, 7.3
Orthopedic Surgeons	"		5.9, 7.1, 7.2, 7.3
Psychiatrists	"		5.10, 7.2
Radiologists	"		5.11, 7.1, 7.2, 7.3
Urologists	"		5.12, 7.1, 7.2, 7.3
Resident Physicians	Physicians in Training in all Specialties per 100,000 persons in HRRs	Price Index for total population	5.13

TABLE TWO

Clinically Active Physician Workforce Serving Residents of Hospital Referral Regions

(Physicians per 100,000 Residents, 1993)*

Hospital Referral Region	Resident Population	All Physicians	Primary Care Physicians	Specialists	Anesthesiologists	Cardiologists	General Surgeons	Obstetrician/ Gynecologists	Ophthalmologists	Orthopedic Surgeons	Psychiatrists	Radiologists	Urologists	Resident Physicians
Alabama														
Birmingham	1,983,947	154.9	55.4	98.2	7.5	4.8	10.0	10.2	4.3	5.8	6.4	8.2	3.2	35.9
Dothan	328,197	137.6	52.1	84.4	6.1	3.5	9.4	10.5	5.6	6.0	4.6	5.9	3.3	9.6
Huntsville	472,826	138.4	52.6	85.5	7.1	2.7	8.5	10.8	2.9	5.8	6.0	6.3	2.9	15.5
Mobile	680,935	160.0	52.3	106.5	8.0	4.0	10.5	14.2	4.6	7.5	7.1	8.2	2.8	33.7
Montgomery	398,081	139.4	49.1	89.6	5.8	3.7	11.2	10.7	4.5	5.6	5.5	5.8	3.3	8.8
Tuscaloosa	228,294	148.3	55.4	90.6	5.0	3.3	9.4	8.5	3.7	5.1	11.8	7.5	2.8	22.7
Alaska														
Anchorage	546,182	183.0	76.0	105.4	8.0	3.7	10.0	8.7	7.0	10.8	10.6	6.7	3.1	12.2
Arizona														
Mesa	683,368	145.5	50.2	94.1	10.1	4.5	7.1	10.8	5.1	5.7	7.2	6.2	2.7	17.6
Phoenix	1,937,465	188.5	63.1	124.3	12.3	5.8	8.6	12.3	6.0	8.0	10.7	8.8	2.7	24.9
Sun City	133,419	256.2	80.0	174.5	16.9	5.2	13.1	25.6	8.9	15.2	13.2	11.4	3.5	25.0
Tucson	838,882	205.1	66.7	136.8	12.4	5.3	9.6	13.4	6.2	8.5	14.5	10.8	3.0	44.1
Arkansas														
Fort Smith	303,027	137.6	55.4	80.6	9.0	4.5	7.9	8.5	3.0	6.3	3.0	6.7	3.1	8.3
Jonesboro	200,076	130.0	53.2	75.8	5.3	2.9	8.0	8.8	3.5	5.3	4.8	7.0	3.4	14.2
Little Rock	1,321,705	159.8	58.7	99.0	7.4	3.9	8.6	9.5	5.5	6.7	9.3	8.0	2.8	34.8
Springdale	295,913	151.2	60.5	90.0	6.6	2.9	10.1	8.0	4.7	6.8	8.6	8.6	3.5	13.1
Texarkana	245,516	129.7	48.6	80.7	6.8	2.9	6.8	11.2	4.0	5.2	5.1	8.7	2.7	9.5
California														
Orange Co.	2,561,917	215.2	71.8	141.3	13.0	7.6	9.5	14.2	6.9	10.2	12.3	9.6	3.4	26.2
Bakersfield	753,777	154.7	55.4	98.2	9.8	4.5	8.0	11.4	6.6	6.8	6.1	7.2	2.8	15.2
Chico	247,777	182.3	59.5	122.0	11.4	4.0	9.5	13.4	6.4	9.5	7.8	11.3	3.6	9.0
Contra Costa Co.	776,882	232.0	76.2	153.8	12.7	5.8	11.7	16.0	7.4	8.9	16.5	11.9	4.4	27.2
Fresno	870,093	159.3	57.3	100.6	10.0	4.8	10.6	9.9	5.7	5.7	8.3	7.9	2.3	20.4
Los Angeles	8,891,233	209.5	70.9	136.2	10.9	7.6	9.2	12.1	6.9	7.8	15.7	9.0	3.6	36.2
Modesto	642,363	161.2	56.9	103.0	10.8	4.6	9.5	11.4	5.2	7.2	6.3	7.7	2.8	13.9
Napa	237,369	264.3	90.9	170.8	12.7	5.4	16.0	17.7	7.6	12.4	29.7	15.7	4.2	14.5
Alameda Co.	1,307,511	244.2	86.8	154.9	10.3	6.3	9.6	14.0	7.7	8.9	20.4	11.2	3.6	31.7
Palm Spr/Rancho Mir.	214,236	229.4	63.7	163.6	15.0	6.9	10.1	18.9	5.4	13.5	14.4	12.5	3.9	22.0
Redding	291,627	199.9	75.4	121.1	12.4	2.4	9.2	11.0	6.6	10.9	7.8	11.1	3.9	12.0
Sacramento	1,826,537	193.8	68.0	123.8	11.2	5.1	8.5	12.9	6.5	9.1	11.1	8.9	3.1	29.0
Salinas	340,435	186.7	59.5	126.2	9.5	5.3	10.8	11.6	8.4	9.8	12.3	8.4	4.6	18.4
San Bernardino	2,052,460	157.6	55.0	101.0	8.8	4.7	8.4	10.5	4.9	7.1	8.8	7.2	3.0	25.5
San Diego	2,767,527	206.0	65.3	138.1	12.9	6.3	8.1	11.6	7.4	9.4	14.9	8.8	3.9	32.0
San Francisco	1,281,325	317.2	116.6	196.8	13.1	8.9	11.4	12.6	8.3	10.7	38.4	14.2	3.6	65.3
San Jose	1,463,526	200.4	71.0	127.1	9.3	7.2	8.9	14.6	6.8	8.4	12.8	7.5	3.5	28.3
San Luis Obispo	205,889	242.4	82.2	159.0	13.0	5.9	11.2	12.8	8.1	11.9	29.3	13.3	3.0	7.4

Hospital Referral Region	Resident Population	All Physicians	Primary Care Physicians	Specialists	Anesthesiologists	Cardiologists	General Surgeons	Obstetrician/ Gynecologists	Ophthalmologists	Orthopedic Surgeons	Psychiatrists	Radiologists	Urologists	Resident Physicians
San Mateo Co.	723,533	241.9	79.6	160.1	11.2	8.2	9.0	12.9	7.2	8.4	26.7	10.7	2.9	49.9
Santa Barbara	374,609	219.9	72.3	146.3	12.2	7.3	11.3	11.9	7.4	10.6	16.4	10.9	4.1	15.2
Santa Cruz	240,944	209.6	64.5	142.7	13.9	4.9	8.3	14.9	7.1	9.5	14.3	8.0	5.0	12.0
Santa Rosa	393,669	241.3	93.6	145.5	12.9	5.7	9.0	13.2	7.8	12.3	19.5	10.5	4.1	19.2
Stockton	413,152	159.3	56.6	101.1	10.1	6.7	7.9	11.9	5.1	7.3	7.9	6.9	2.5	15.3
Ventura	700,513	200.3	68.1	130.3	11.2	6.2	8.7	12.1	7.1	9.9	15.3	7.8	3.7	14.9
Colorado														
Boulder	212,469	217.7	77.4	139.0	12.5	3.8	8.3	11.9	8.3	9.5	19.8	6.6	2.9	16.7
Colorado Springs	561,723	180.5	63.1	116.4	8.7	4.6	10.5	11.0	6.6	9.9	10.8	7.3	3.4	11.2
Denver	1,904,201	217.6	74.6	141.3	11.6	6.2	8.5	13.0	7.6	9.1	16.5	9.8	3.1	49.0
Fort Collins	238,089	170.2	63.3	106.5	9.7	4.9	8.4	8.6	8.7	8.1	8.8	6.9	4.4	15.7
Grand Junction	201,585	187.1	75.5	109.6	14.1	1.7	11.0	8.0	6.5	12.5	7.6	8.4	3.4	12.6
Greeley	227,007	181.5	67.2	113.6	10.8	3.5	12.0	12.0	7.3	9.9	6.5	7.3	4.1	17.5
Pueblo	133,475	186.7	68.1	117.8	8.9	3.2	9.3	11.2	7.3	9.8	13.2	6.2	2.6	15.7
Connecticut														
Bridgeport	629,535	239.1	75.4	162.3	10.7	6.1	10.5	18.3	8.9	9.3	22.5	10.5	3.9	44.5
Hartford	1,393,087	214.7	67.6	145.2	11.6	6.9	9.9	14.8	6.7	9.0	22.3	11.0	3.3	45.6
New Haven	1,349,858	231.2	73.8	155.4	10.9	7.0	10.3	14.2	7.5	8.9	25.2	10.7	3.4	61.0
Delaware														
Wilmington	635,637	198.2	69.6	127.4	7.9	6.4	10.3	11.2	6.1	6.6	14.3	10.2	3.1	33.9
District of Columbia														
Washington	2,153,979	291.1	89.6	198.9	12.7	9.2	12.6	17.5	9.6	8.7	29.5	12.5	5.0	68.7
Florida														
Bradenton	197,705	167.6	48.3	117.3	10.5	6.0	8.2	15.1	4.7	6.5	9.1	8.3	2.5	12.1
Clearwater	450,255	192.5	64.4	126.7	9.5	4.3	7.0	13.9	5.0	8.1	11.8	11.7	2.8	19.2
Fort Lauderdale	1,927,706	227.8	72.4	154.0	11.8	7.2	9.9	18.8	7.2	9.8	13.0	10.6	4.2	18.5
Fort Myers	627,321	191.3	58.9	131.0	10.4	4.8	9.3	18.4	5.7	8.1	9.9	10.8	3.1	12.5
Gainesville	407,508	201.8	66.1	133.0	12.6	6.4	9.0	9.7	5.0	7.0	13.7	11.5	3.6	92.6
Hudson	287,224	181.1	60.5	119.3	8.4	5.5	8.2	15.5	4.8	8.6	10.1	9.5	3.2	18.4
Jacksonville	1,137,244	186.0	62.2	122.5	10.7	7.5	9.7	11.8	5.6	6.9	8.8	9.0	3.8	29.2
Lakeland	279,997	139.3	46.1	92.2	8.4	4.5	7.9	11.3	4.3	5.1	6.8	6.5	2.4	12.2
Miami	2,365,502	237.8	83.0	151.5	11.3	10.1	11.4	13.9	7.9	7.4	16.7	9.9	4.2	42.7
Ocala	292,949	163.9	47.4	115.0	10.0	4.8	8.3	14.3	4.0	6.5	10.9	11.4	3.2	21.6
Orlando	2,251,255	169.1	56.6	111.4	9.9	5.4	8.2	13.6	5.1	8.2	7.6	8.8	3.8	15.0
Ormond Beach	268,338	162.4	56.9	104.4	8.6	3.5	7.4	11.0	5.4	9.5	8.6	9.4	2.9	13.6
Panama City	161,325	149.2	53.1	95.4	6.0	3.0	10.1	10.7	5.3	5.6	7.7	7.0	4.2	7.3
Pensacola	588,018	170.1	54.7	114.2	9.5	4.2	10.6	11.9	6.3	7.3	8.6	9.6	2.6	24.4
Sarasota	317,728	216.5	65.3	149.3	13.2	6.5	9.2	17.5	6.9	9.7	15.2	11.3	4.3	13.9
St Petersburg	401,404	201.1	67.2	132.3	10.9	5.5	7.8	13.8	5.2	8.2	9.8	11.8	3.0	27.5
Tallahassee	628,832	152.2	56.9	94.4	7.7	3.3	9.6	9.6	4.9	5.1	10.3	7.3	3.2	11.6
Tampa	876,408	185.1	60.4	123.3	9.2	6.4	7.3	11.5	5.9	6.7	12.2	9.8	3.3	38.4
Georgia														
Albany	200,455	120.3	39.1	80.2	5.7	2.7	7.4	11.2	3.3	5.1	5.2	7.0	3.4	6.8
Atlanta	3,700,835	178.7	58.3	119.3	10.2	6.0	9.3	13.7	5.8	7.1	10.5	8.1	4.0	28.1
Augusta	548,493	201.5	64.9	134.5	8.1	6.7	11.0	12.8	4.9	6.2	16.3	10.3	3.4	72.6
Columbus	301,665	137.7	49.6	86.8	6.5	3.4	6.8	9.6	3.7	9.2	9.2	7.1	3.0	21.9

Hospital Referral Region	Resident Population	All Physicians	Primary Care Physicians	Specialists	Anesthesiologists	Cardiologists	General Surgeons	Obstetrician/ Gynecologists	Ophthalmologists	Orthopedic Surgeons	Psychiatrists	Radiologists	Urologists	Resident Physicians
Macon	597,635	164.1	56.2	106.4	9.8	3.1	11.6	14.0	5.1	6.4	8.9	8.3	3.4	21.2
Rome	220,157	151.5	59.1	90.9	8.1	3.6	10.2	13.3	4.3	4.6	5.0	8.2	3.3	19.0
Savannah	601,416	158.1	53.2	103.8	8.3	3.4	11.5	14.3	4.8	6.5	8.0	7.6	3.8	22.7
Hawaii														
Honolulu	1,108,229	214.2	77.7	134.6	10.1	5.1	11.4	14.7	7.6	7.1	15.9	8.6	3.2	38.2
Idaho														
Boise	517,555	160.8	54.3	106.0	8.3	2.9	9.9	10.9	5.4	9.2	8.4	8.0	3.5	14.8
Idaho Falls	166,131	131.3	41.7	87.9	9.0	3.3	9.8	11.2	5.5	7.9	6.1	6.0	1.8	8.4
Illinois														
Aurora	181,602	137.4	49.5	87.7	6.4	4.0	10.3	8.3	5.0	8.1	5.5	5.2	3.7	11.9
Blue Island	805,400	182.1	64.3	115.9	11.2	6.9	10.4	14.3	5.1	6.6	8.7	7.9	2.7	37.1
Chicago	2,680,712	227.5	85.9	139.3	9.6	8.2	10.1	13.3	6.0	5.5	20.0	8.9	2.8	98.7
Elgin	522,152	151.0	53.0	96.4	10.1	4.5	8.2	10.3	6.6	6.1	8.5	4.7	3.0	17.9
Evanston	861,134	245.9	84.3	159.4	15.2	7.3	10.0	18.3	7.1	9.2	18.3	11.9	3.7	51.8
Hinsdale	341,601	219.7	73.9	143.9	20.4	7.6	8.9	12.2	5.9	5.9	11.6	12.7	4.1	41.9
Joliet	438,832	152.2	52.5	98.9	10.7	4.7	10.0	12.4	4.2	5.4	7.8	6.1	2.7	17.9
Melrose Park	1,189,327	213.8	77.9	133.9	11.7	7.2	9.9	14.3	6.7	6.9	11.1	8.6	3.6	63.7
Peoria	601,129	147.9	50.3	97.0	8.8	4.7	8.5	9.9	3.7	5.0	5.9	9.0	2.9	22.9
Rockford	623,702	153.1	54.3	98.0	10.1	4.3	8.7	10.3	4.9	6.3	7.0	6.7	3.0	13.2
Springfield	820,868	137.2	50.5	85.7	7.2	3.5	8.4	8.6	4.2	4.9	5.5	7.7	2.5	22.0
Urbana	429,114	147.0	56.2	90.4	6.9	3.9	8.4	8.3	3.6	5.0	9.2	6.4	3.0	17.1
Bloomington	163,421	139.6	48.8	90.6	8.6	4.7	9.1	7.6	7.0	4.3	4.8	7.4	2.3	9.1
Indiana														
Evansville	646,627	135.3	53.7	80.8	7.8	3.7	7.4	8.3	2.9	5.4	6.4	6.8	2.8	9.4
Fort Wayne	767,226	126.1	48.5	76.8	7.7	4.1	8.3	6.4	3.7	5.8	4.8	7.6	2.5	9.0
Gary	485,735	148.6	52.9	94.6	9.3	5.4	8.5	9.4	4.6	5.3	6.0	8.3	2.1	10.4
Indianapolis	2,324,142	164.7	59.2	104.8	10.8	5.4	8.3	9.2	4.6	6.2	9.0	8.1	2.8	39.4
Lafayette	197,673	139.3	49.9	87.7	10.5	3.9	5.7	6.7	3.9	5.2	7.7	5.9	2.2	11.5
Muncie	171,507	138.8	50.4	87.2	10.4	2.7	7.4	6.9	4.6	6.1	4.1	6.5	3.0	27.6
Munster	296,292	162.9	56.7	104.8	9.2	4.6	10.1	12.1	5.6	6.2	7.0	8.0	2.8	16.5
South Bend	611,180	141.2	54.3	86.4	10.2	2.7	8.4	8.7	3.9	5.7	6.4	7.3	2.5	12.6
Terre Haute	176,806	134.1	50.2	83.6	9.7	3.6	8.0	9.2	5.0	4.9	7.3	6.1	3.3	16.1
Iowa														
Cedar Rapids	252,695	141.3	53.1	87.8	9.2	2.6	5.7	6.1	4.7	7.3	8.9	7.0	2.2	24.8
Davenport	486,583	148.4	52.6	94.7	9.0	3.1	8.5	10.5	6.3	6.6	6.4	7.1	2.7	21.4
Des Moines	928,747	150.2	61.7	87.8	9.0	3.9	8.5	7.9	4.1	5.1	5.9	7.3	2.3	20.7
Dubuque	147,879	141.8	50.3	90.8	5.0	2.4	8.7	7.9	6.8	6.8	5.0	7.4	2.6	16.9
Iowa City	308,514	169.1	59.0	109.3	9.7	4.7	7.9	9.0	5.7	5.5	8.4	10.5	3.1	107.8
Mason City	143,369	140.2	63.0	76.3	5.6	2.8	8.0	6.8	3.5	6.3	5.6	6.9	2.6	28.2
Sioux City	252,103	119.0	49.7	68.1	5.6	3.1	7.7	5.4	2.7	5.0	7.1	5.1	2.7	18.2
Waterloo	205,443	142.6	57.4	85.0	10.3	2.9	7.3	7.8	4.3	5.7	8.3	5.5	2.5	25.5
Kansas														
Topeka	421,682	154.3	54.2	99.0	5.1	3.4	6.8	8.2	4.2	5.9	21.7	7.9	2.8	17.1
Wichita	1,169,518	142.9	62.0	80.2	6.7	3.5	8.8	7.8	3.5	5.4	6.8	7.8	2.6	20.3
Kentucky														
Covington	316,933	154.6	57.3	96.6	9.2	2.8	7.7	13.2	3.5	6.7	9.2	6.4	3.4	33.5

Hospital Referral Region	Resident Population	All Physicians	Primary Care Physicians	Specialists	Anesthesiologists	Cardiologists	General Surgeons	Obstetrician/ Gynecologists	Ophthalmologists	Orthopedic Surgeons	Psychiatrists	Radiologists	Urologists	Resident Physicians
Lexington	1,290,244	155.5	60.4	93.6	7.2	4.2	9.6	9.4	4.6	4.7	8.7	7.9	3.1	33.0
Louisville	1,464,748	167.6	59.8	106.4	10.9	4.6	10.4	10.0	4.6	6.4	10.4	8.0	2.9	32.6
Owensboro	131,949	132.4	46.5	85.8	8.8	3.7	10.0	8.6	3.5	6.5	5.6	5.8	3.8	8.4
Paducah	342,954	129.8	46.4	82.4	5.5	2.4	9.6	11.0	3.6	5.5	3.4	8.2	3.2	13.4
Louisiana														
Alexandria	277,018	142.6	50.1	90.7	6.0	5.1	11.5	10.8	5.7	5.5	8.8	5.0	3.4	12.6
Baton Rouge	734,846	152.3	55.2	96.8	7.1	4.5	9.0	11.3	6.2	5.8	6.1	6.0	3.3	15.3
Houma	245,201	122.9	36.3	85.9	5.4	6.7	11.3	10.4	4.6	6.6	4.5	4.5	5.0	15.2
Lafayette	535,796	136.4	49.8	85.7	6.6	2.9	9.4	11.4	5.1	5.8	4.6	7.1	3.4	9.1
Lake Charles	258,157	121.5	41.8	78.9	3.9	4.0	6.6	12.0	4.8	6.5	3.3	6.8	2.7	12.9
Metairie	396,726	231.3	65.8	164.7	12.3	7.1	14.2	19.7	11.1	7.4	16.0	10.8	4.7	67.7
Monroe	266,139	133.3	48.5	83.3	7.3	2.1	7.7	9.6	3.6	5.5	4.3	6.6	3.1	8.9
New Orleans	838,284	223.8	61.1	161.0	9.6	8.4	11.9	13.7	8.5	9.5	19.1	12.1	4.5	76.7
Shreveport	646,435	151.1	49.4	100.6	8.9	4.7	9.2	11.5	4.6	6.8	5.9	7.2	3.8	38.8
Slidell	140,609	162.7	47.5	114.8	12.9	5.0	10.4	15.6	6.3	7.5	9.2	7.1	3.6	20.3
Maine														
Bangor	396,634	169.8	69.0	100.4	7.8	3.3	11.4	10.5	5.3	7.6	9.3	7.9	2.5	12.6
Portland	948,869	197.4	72.6	124.2	9.2	5.1	10.7	11.7	5.2	10.0	13.9	9.0	2.6	22.8
Maryland														
Baltimore	2,247,761	251.0	82.6	166.9	13.0	8.0	13.5	17.7	7.7	8.3	22.1	11.3	3.5	78.4
Salisbury	305,907	181.9	60.8	120.5	10.3	6.4	12.0	14.4	6.5	8.2	9.3	8.9	3.6	15.7
Takoma Park	778,169	268.7	89.4	175.6	11.7	9.6	13.1	17.7	8.7	7.9	20.3	11.2	5.4	94.0
Massachusetts														
Boston	4,418,982	256.0	82.9	171.0	12.0	8.2	11.3	14.0	6.9	8.7	30.5	13.0	3.1	77.1
Springfield	727,784	193.7	67.3	125.5	10.7	5.9	11.2	12.0	5.6	7.1	16.0	9.4	2.9	30.7
Worcester	711,982	210.7	79.9	129.3	10.3	7.8	9.0	11.1	5.2	7.6	14.6	9.0	3.3	62.6
Michigan														
Ann Arbor	1,192,620	195.0	66.6	126.9	8.0	7.1	9.1	10.7	5.8	4.9	18.6	10.6	3.5	78.8
Dearborn	524,139	174.9	64.2	109.6	7.6	4.8	9.0	14.7	6.2	5.8	9.1	8.7	3.1	56.5
Detroit	1,937,050	176.2	61.7	113.4	6.9	5.7	9.7	12.7	5.3	5.2	9.7	9.0	2.5	61.4
Flint	550,338	159.0	70.0	87.3	7.9	4.6	9.8	8.0	4.9	3.4	5.9	8.2	2.5	47.2
Grand Rapids	954,534	147.7	54.6	92.5	7.6	2.6	8.9	10.0	4.8	6.5	7.2	6.9	2.9	32.8
Kalamazoo	620,043	165.8	61.3	103.3	7.0	4.7	10.3	9.7	4.5	6.1	11.0	7.1	2.6	19.0
Lansing	647,965	165.4	65.8	98.4	7.9	5.0	7.6	9.5	4.4	6.4	9.1	7.6	2.7	41.5
Marquette	202,537	157.1	61.1	95.3	5.5	3.8	11.4	11.6	4.4	5.7	6.4	7.8	2.4	18.3
Muskegon	241,421	155.0	60.4	94.1	8.2	3.1	6.8	8.1	4.8	7.1	6.6	7.3	3.4	14.2
Petoskey	148,605	165.8	64.9	99.6	8.0	3.5	11.0	8.9	4.1	7.2	6.5	8.0	3.5	10.9
Pontiac	391,240	204.1	69.2	134.1	10.8	6.4	11.1	13.2	5.6	5.1	18.0	11.1	2.8	58.2
Royal Oak	650,771	254.2	88.3	164.6	9.1	7.7	10.2	17.0	7.5	6.9	22.8	14.0	3.2	88.5
Saginaw	628,840	148.7	58.7	89.2	8.9	3.8	9.4	9.5	4.5	5.0	5.3	8.1	2.9	21.2
St Joseph	145,896	155.6	55.1	98.4	9.2	7.4	12.1	10.1	4.9	6.2	8.0	9.2	2.0	12.3
Traverse City	177,508	192.0	71.9	119.2	9.1	3.6	11.7	11.0	5.0	7.4	12.6	11.7	2.9	14.7
Minnesota														
Duluth	323,298	165.9	71.4	93.0	6.3	2.7	8.9	8.2	4.9	6.3	7.3	6.8	2.8	17.3
Minneapolis	2,614,660	172.6	70.9	100.6	7.6	4.1	7.8	8.9	5.5	7.0	9.5	7.5	2.6	33.9
Rochester	363,251	218.7	78.3	139.7	8.0	12.0	7.5	7.6	4.7	6.4	9.4	11.8	2.3	113.0

Hospital Referral Region	Resident Population	All Physicians	Primary Care Physicians	Specialists	Anesthesiologists	Cardiologists	General Surgeons	Obstetrician/ Gynecologists	Ophthalmologists	Orthopedic Surgeons	Psychiatrists	Radiologists	Urologists	Resident Physicians
St Cloud	205,700	142.2	62.8	77.6	7.7	3.0	8.0	8.5	3.8	5.7	6.6	4.6	3.2	10.3
St Paul	840,098	183.1	78.5	102.8	6.2	4.7	8.8	8.9	6.5	7.4	10.3	8.2	2.1	39.7
Mississippi														
Gulfport	175,723	170.3	48.8	120.4	7.7	3.3	11.3	12.5	7.2	7.8	11.0	9.2	3.7	38.3
Hattiesburg	252,292	137.0	47.4	88.5	8.3	4.1	8.5	9.3	5.3	6.6	4.6	6.4	2.9	8.4
Jackson	979,993	143.4	51.6	90.7	8.1	3.2	7.2	9.2	5.0	5.4	7.4	7.2	2.9	29.5
Meridian	192,396	132.8	52.2	79.8	4.9	3.5	8.5	9.7	4.6	4.8	7.2	5.2	3.0	10.7
Oxford	129,317	129.6	51.0	77.5	6.8	3.5	9.3	11.4	5.4	4.3	2.8	5.8	3.4	15.0
Tupelo	349,277	113.6	44.9	67.6	4.9	2.0	9.9	9.6	2.9	4.1	2.5	5.4	2.6	9.1
Missouri														
Cape Girardeau	253,402	130.1	49.9	79.7	7.1	3.4	9.3	9.0	3.6	3.2	5.4	6.7	3.0	12.0
Columbia	587,088	168.7	62.3	105.5	8.7	4.8	8.8	9.9	4.1	6.7	9.8	8.5	2.6	56.0
Joplin	311,296	138.7	56.3	82.1	5.3	3.1	8.4	11.6	4.1	5.8	5.7	7.2	2.8	9.2
Kansas City	2,025,703	178.4	65.0	112.5	9.2	4.7	8.1	10.5	5.8	6.7	11.2	8.5	2.9	36.4
Springfield	619,065	142.1	54.2	87.2	7.0	3.0	9.2	8.2	3.8	5.9	5.9	6.6	2.7	9.1
St Louis	3,134,871	178.7	62.8	114.2	8.6	5.6	9.8	12.4	5.7	6.3	10.4	10.1	2.8	49.0
Montana														
Billings	463,221	173.5	64.0	108.8	10.7	3.5	11.9	10.3	5.2	10.2	10.6	7.6	3.0	6.6
Great Falls	148,937	167.3	60.3	106.2	11.0	2.8	8.2	10.3	4.9	10.0	6.8	8.5	2.9	10.8
Missoula	288,550	200.4	71.9	127.7	13.3	4.8	11.9	10.8	6.7	12.1	8.7	7.8	3.6	6.6
Nebraska														
Lincoln	508,894	135.1	57.9	76.9	6.3	2.7	8.7	7.2	4.0	5.7	6.7	6.2	2.7	12.0
Omaha	1,119,894	157.4	57.4	99.4	7.3	5.9	9.3	8.7	4.8	5.9	8.3	9.2	2.4	40.1
Nevada														
Las Vegas	794,033	167.0	54.8	111.0	11.8	6.8	8.3	11.9	4.6	6.1	6.2	9.0	3.0	15.2
Reno	483,100	188.7	63.4	122.7	13.0	6.0	11.8	11.4	6.1	8.6	7.7	9.1	3.6	16.1
New Hampshire														
Lebanon	363,701	205.8	76.1	128.7	11.0	5.3	11.2	10.6	5.4	7.3	22.1	8.7	2.7	56.7
Manchester	740,593	180.9	60.5	119.7	8.8	6.5	8.8	12.4	5.6	9.6	15.6	7.4	3.5	11.9
New Jersey														
Camden	2,454,954	208.6	70.7	136.8	10.3	8.2	11.6	16.0	6.1	8.0	12.7	10.2	3.9	44.8
Hackensack	1,129,751	266.0	90.0	174.3	16.0	9.3	12.4	18.0	8.8	8.5	24.1	10.9	4.5	65.6
Morristown	878,642	229.8	76.5	152.4	12.1	8.7	11.4	16.8	7.4	8.6	16.7	11.3	4.3	39.1
New Brunswick	838,495	226.2	80.4	144.3	10.9	9.3	10.7	15.5	6.6	8.2	17.1	8.8	3.6	61.0
Newark	1,466,813	212.3	76.9	134.1	9.6	7.7	10.2	14.8	7.1	6.8	12.4	8.5	4.2	57.8
Paterson	364,246	179.3	67.7	111.0	7.7	6.0	10.0	13.3	6.3	6.2	10.2	7.2	3.9	40.6
Ridgewood	379,311	226.7	73.6	152.1	14.0	9.4	11.4	16.7	8.2	8.8	22.3	8.4	4.4	31.3
New Mexico														
Albuquerque	1,254,781	198.3	74.3	122.7	10.4	4.7	10.5	11.8	6.4	8.5	13.4	8.2	3.3	33.5
New York														
Albany	1,721,696	197.9	66.0	130.8	10.0	5.9	10.8	12.6	6.3	6.9	16.5	9.8	3.8	28.5
Binghamton	376,954	164.0	54.9	108.3	8.8	4.7	10.6	12.3	4.4	7.8	12.5	8.8	3.1	19.8
Bronx	1,211,361	213.2	74.4	137.5	8.1	7.3	9.8	11.7	5.8	3.9	24.5	8.5	3.6	97.6
Buffalo	1,437,600	179.1	60.3	117.8	9.5	4.9	12.9	12.7	5.6	5.6	10.0	9.8	3.4	39.6
Elmira	344,696	181.0	56.8	123.5	10.7	4.2	11.8	14.8	4.7	7.9	15.8	9.1	3.5	13.6
East Long Island	4,242,448	265.0	92.3	171.0	13.4	7.7	12.6	18.7	8.7	7.8	25.8	11.3	4.1	76.8

Hospital Referral Region	Resident Population	All Physicians	Primary Care Physicians	Specialists	Anesthesiologists	Cardiologists	General Surgeons	Obstetrician/ Gynecologists	Ophthalmologists	Orthopedic Surgeons	Psychiatrists	Radiologists	Urologists	Resident Physicians
New York	4,568,777	265.7	88.6	175.6	9.9	9.3	12.1	14.1	8.5	5.7	35.5	10.5	4.1	111.1
Rochester	1,243,904	185.0	70.0	113.9	9.9	4.6	9.3	13.2	6.3	6.5	14.7	8.9	2.9	53.4
Syracuse	1,074,023	163.4	56.0	106.5	9.6	5.1	9.2	11.5	5.4	7.5	11.3	8.8	3.4	38.5
White Plains	1,025,646	303.8	93.7	208.6	15.7	8.4	14.4	19.7	10.9	8.9	43.9	13.4	4.9	74.2
North Carolina														
Asheville	490,407	177.5	68.9	107.9	8.4	2.5	9.6	10.1	4.7	8.8	10.5	9.2	4.0	12.3
Charlotte	1,558,895	149.0	50.3	98.0	6.4	4.0	8.8	12.5	5.3	6.9	6.9	7.8	3.8	18.7
Durham	1,044,489	189.9	59.5	129.0	9.4	5.6	8.7	11.4	5.4	7.0	17.6	12.1	4.0	87.4
Greensboro	473,708	157.1	54.3	102.3	7.1	5.0	7.6	11.4	6.3	6.8	7.3	8.3	3.7	23.4
Greenville	696,239	153.9	52.7	99.9	6.2	4.8	10.4	12.8	4.9	6.5	8.2	7.5	2.9	41.3
Hickory	236,085	124.9	44.8	79.2	5.4	2.9	9.0	10.8	3.3	5.7	4.5	7.5	3.3	10.4
Raleigh	1,279,158	154.9	55.8	98.1	5.5	4.7	8.8	10.2	4.7	5.3	12.0	7.4	3.6	27.3
Wilmington	277,569	175.2	57.0	117.4	9.0	4.0	11.6	13.9	5.6	8.1	8.3	8.7	4.0	28.5
Winston-Salem	883,657	146.9	49.4	96.9	7.7	4.5	8.3	10.6	4.1	5.3	8.5	8.5	3.1	41.0
North Dakota														
Bismarck	201,983	150.9	54.6	96.1	12.0	3.8	9.3	8.7	3.5	4.9	4.7	7.5	2.7	14.2
Fargo Moorhead -Mn	464,935	145.7	63.8	80.9	4.8	2.8	8.3	7.0	5.1	5.6	10.5	6.4	2.2	18.1
Grand Forks	179,647	136.7	62.5	71.5	4.7	1.8	8.3	6.5	3.3	6.5	4.2	4.5	2.2	32.9
Minot	127,785	149.3	57.5	91.5	8.2	2.1	9.5	9.3	4.0	6.9	7.9	9.1	3.9	22.0
Ohio														
Akron	668,249	182.1	67.2	112.9	8.5	4.3	9.6	11.4	4.8	8.7	8.2	8.1	3.2	52.6
Canton	602,501	139.9	52.4	86.5	7.7	3.4	7.9	10.8	5.1	6.2	5.2	6.9	2.4	23.7
Cincinnati	1,509,444	190.6	66.0	123.7	10.1	5.3	8.9	12.9	5.2	7.3	13.8	8.2	3.2	46.3
Cleveland	2,086,998	213.0	71.2	140.5	12.9	7.3	11.3	12.4	6.3	7.4	12.7	12.0	2.7	70.8
Columbus	2,525,830	153.6	57.1	95.5	8.4	4.6	8.2	9.5	4.7	6.0	8.1	6.7	2.9	33.8
Dayton	1,111,678	147.4	56.9	89.8	7.4	4.2	8.6	9.1	3.5	5.3	5.5	6.7	2.9	26.2
Elyria	241,159	152.8	57.5	94.6	9.4	4.9	8.7	9.3	3.9	6.3	6.3	8.0	2.9	19.0
Kettering	360,768	189.6	69.0	119.3	11.1	4.4	7.4	10.4	6.1	7.2	9.1	10.1	3.7	47.1
Toledo	982,485	172.9	61.2	111.3	11.1	4.8	10.2	11.6	5.4	6.3	7.0	8.5	3.7	37.3
Youngstown	688,740	168.6	65.2	102.9	9.2	3.9	11.4	10.8	4.2	6.1	6.8	10.5	2.4	32.6
Oklahoma														
Lawton	192,373	138.5	56.4	80.8	5.4	2.4	8.3	7.9	3.0	5.8	7.9	7.3	3.1	18.0
Oklahoma City	1,565,094	162.3	60.0	100.4	8.7	5.0	8.8	9.6	4.5	6.2	9.0	8.0	3.5	31.6
Tulsa	1,140,749	159.6	62.5	96.1	8.6	5.2	8.4	10.4	4.4	6.1	7.0	8.1	3.0	22.2
Oregon														
Bend	121,666	170.0	61.4	107.6	11.0	2.6	10.2	11.9	6.6	5.9	6.4	10.1	4.8	6.6
Eugene	604,042	179.7	68.3	110.3	10.8	2.7	8.9	11.7	6.1	9.7	8.8	6.5	3.1	6.7
Medford	338,364	180.1	67.0	111.4	9.2	3.5	9.0	12.1	6.6	12.1	7.0	8.5	3.8	7.6
Portland	1,894,661	202.4	71.2	130.2	12.5	5.2	9.1	13.3	6.6	8.3	12.3	9.1	3.3	30.0
Salem	227,361	181.8	63.8	115.9	11.3	2.2	9.9	10.8	7.7	9.6	11.9	8.9	3.1	7.8
Pennsylvania														
Allentown	985,564	180.5	65.7	113.8	9.5	6.5	10.1	11.7	5.7	6.9	8.9	9.4	3.3	23.9
Altoona	297,507	147.0	54.2	92.5	6.9	3.8	8.4	11.2	3.8	5.9	5.5	9.1	2.5	17.2
Danville	536,017	169.0	58.9	109.2	8.7	4.8	8.7	8.0	4.6	5.8	6.8	11.0	2.9	28.8
Erie	732,505	154.8	53.7	100.5	7.5	3.6	11.4	9.1	4.5	7.7	7.6	9.0	3.2	16.8
Harrisburg	879,941	167.6	65.4	101.4	9.0	4.3	7.8	10.9	4.7	7.1	8.4	8.9	3.2	37.0

Hospital Referral Region	Resident Population	All Physicians	Primary Care Physicians	Specialists	Anesthesiologists	Cardiologists	General Surgeons	Obstetrician/ Gynecologists	Ophthalmologists	Orthopedic Surgeons	Psychiatrists	Radiologists	Urologists	Resident Physicians
Johnstown	241,968	163.0	61.2	100.2	9.0	3.9	9.2	11.9	4.5	5.7	6.4	9.5	3.0	36.8
Lancaster	529,921	160.1	61.9	97.7	9.5	6.1	6.4	8.3	5.3	6.6	8.4	9.1	2.9	20.1
Philadelphia	3,921,220	259.4	89.3	168.5	10.8	9.8	10.5	14.9	7.1	7.8	24.7	13.6	3.6	77.8
Pittsburgh	3,055,252	186.3	62.9	122.4	10.1	6.2	10.3	11.5	4.8	6.1	11.4	11.8	2.8	48.6
Reading	510,057	162.4	62.6	98.9	9.1	3.8	7.9	10.8	5.0	6.5	8.2	9.1	2.8	23.0
Sayre	191,385	148.8	55.0	93.3	7.8	4.4	8.2	7.4	4.3	6.2	5.5	8.0	3.5	18.8
Scranton	300,457	184.1	67.3	116.4	8.4	5.0	11.0	11.0	5.0	6.4	11.7	9.8	2.6	17.5
Wilkes-Barre	258,306	196.0	75.3	120.3	6.5	6.1	9.2	14.0	6.3	4.8	9.0	11.9	5.0	22.1
York	340,946	153.8	62.5	91.1	10.6	3.4	6.6	9.7	4.2	6.3	4.6	7.3	3.5	29.9
Rhode Island														
Providence	1,151,761	197.6	67.8	128.0	8.5	6.2	12.7	12.0	5.4	8.6	15.1	9.8	3.4	48.3
South Carolina														
Charleston	742,214	189.7	60.3	127.7	10.3	4.1	11.2	11.7	7.1	7.3	13.4	8.4	4.7	63.6
Columbia	980,780	157.1	54.6	101.8	7.6	4.6	9.8	10.4	5.8	6.0	13.4	6.8	2.9	29.2
Florence	333,436	130.7	53.7	76.0	6.4	2.4	9.7	10.2	3.4	4.5	4.5	6.5	3.6	17.2
Greenville	682,364	154.5	57.2	96.6	8.7	2.5	9.4	10.7	5.2	7.9	7.3	7.7	3.5	22.1
Spartanburg	306,233	144.9	51.9	92.6	7.2	3.1	13.1	11.2	3.5	7.1	3.6	8.5	3.8	23.3
South Dakota														
Rapid City	184,008	156.8	63.7	91.0	4.2	2.5	12.3	6.3	4.6	5.7	9.2	10.3	2.4	12.8
Sioux Falls	699,852	139.4	62.6	75.8	5.1	2.7	8.5	7.3	4.0	5.9	5.5	6.2	2.9	19.3
Tennessee														
Chattanooga	563,958	160.9	54.3	105.6	10.4	3.4	9.0	11.3	4.5	6.8	8.3	8.5	2.6	17.9
Jackson	287,699	125.4	54.4	70.6	5.1	2.1	8.8	8.8	3.3	4.4	4.5	6.2	3.7	13.2
Johnson City	217,622	188.9	73.9	114.4	8.5	4.0	11.2	12.2	5.1	8.5	8.7	8.1	3.8	46.2
Kingsport	464,124	159.2	63.0	94.9	5.8	3.9	11.8	10.3	3.6	6.6	5.4	8.1	3.2	13.4
Knoxville	1,067,260	160.5	58.6	101.1	8.0	4.7	8.1	11.7	4.2	6.1	7.7	8.8	2.9	15.5
Memphis	1,597,501	150.4	50.7	98.8	8.9	4.5	9.3	10.3	4.2	4.7	7.1	8.2	3.3	34.4
Nashville	1,944,017	166.2	57.2	108.3	8.4	4.3	10.5	11.1	5.3	6.7	8.7	9.5	3.9	35.5
Texas														
Abilene	278,103	146.4	54.9	90.9	7.9	3.8	7.7	11.8	3.9	5.5	5.9	6.7	2.3	12.2
Amarillo	386,240	139.5	50.1	88.5	8.4	4.1	11.4	11.4	3.0	5.5	5.6	6.8	2.7	15.6
Austin	870,567	180.9	65.3	114.7	8.8	4.0	8.1	10.7	6.8	7.6	17.3	6.1	3.3	15.9
Beaumont	425,872	160.9	57.8	102.4	9.7	5.2	8.7	11.1	5.0	6.6	7.0	7.4	4.0	19.5
Bryan	184,248	136.4	56.5	79.2	6.4	3.3	7.1	8.4	4.5	4.9	6.5	7.1	3.0	13.6
Corpus Christi	492,319	156.1	58.7	96.3	11.6	3.6	7.8	10.3	5.3	5.8	5.4	7.3	2.8	19.2
Dallas	3,070,082	170.7	56.2	113.6	11.0	5.3	9.8	12.2	5.9	7.1	9.7	8.0	3.3	35.3
El Paso	811,036	142.0	43.4	96.7	8.4	5.1	8.0	8.9	4.6	7.1	7.1	5.0	2.4	30.4
Fort Worth	1,429,666	154.4	53.9	99.5	9.6	4.0	8.6	11.2	5.1	6.6	6.7	7.2	2.3	18.2
Harlingen	377,065	101.8	35.4	65.5	5.2	2.6	8.0	7.7	5.2	3.5	3.7	4.4	2.4	8.0
Houston	4,195,450	175.2	56.2	117.7	10.3	7.4	8.6	10.8	5.8	6.0	10.3	7.8	3.1	52.1
Longview	182,480	130.5	48.2	81.7	7.6	2.9	6.2	11.2	4.6	5.4	4.4	6.2	3.3	9.5
Lubbock	634,031	153.4	56.5	95.4	9.3	3.8	11.6	9.3	4.7	7.6	6.8	7.5	3.1	29.9
McAllen	324,820	92.5	36.0	56.3	5.9	3.0	5.3	6.8	3.5	3.3	3.4	3.3	1.6	11.8
Odessa	306,783	118.9	39.1	78.7	6.2	2.9	7.7	11.4	4.4	5.6	5.3	4.6	3.2	10.2
San Angelo	150,062	146.6	44.9	101.5	11.7	4.5	9.2	10.4	4.5	7.3	5.7	7.6	3.7	8.7
San Antonio	1,795,095	184.8	57.9	125.1	12.2	4.8	9.4	10.5	6.6	7.1	12.5	8.8	3.2	56.6

Hospital Referral Region	Resident Population	All Physicians	Primary Care Physicians	Specialists	Anesthesiologists	Cardiologists	General Surgeons	Obstetrician/ Gynecologists	Ophthalmologists	Orthopedic Surgeons	Psychiatrists	Radiologists	Urologists	Resident Physicians
Temple	323,119	165.0	60.4	102.9	6.9	5.2	9.0	8.5	6.2	5.5	9.5	8.8	3.2	44.0
Tyler	425,534	159.2	56.5	102.2	9.8	3.1	10.5	11.9	5.4	6.2	7.7	8.2	3.5	13.6
Victoria	133,472	148.6	53.7	93.9	9.4	2.5	7.0	10.2	3.6	5.9	7.7	9.2	2.3	14.2
Waco	279,913	149.8	56.2	92.6	8.9	2.8	7.0	8.8	4.7	6.2	10.9	7.2	3.6	19.9
Wichita Falls	194,271	163.0	56.6	104.0	7.9	2.6	10.3	11.6	3.7	7.2	16.6	8.6	3.0	21.0
Utah														
Ogden	307,965	145.2	46.3	97.6	10.6	3.2	8.6	13.0	5.4	7.1	6.7	6.1	2.5	15.9
Provo	312,598	140.9	48.7	92.1	8.7	2.9	6.3	10.8	5.0	7.0	9.4	5.2	3.2	10.1
Salt Lake City	1,376,597	181.0	56.4	123.9	13.6	5.4	10.2	12.4	5.7	8.9	10.8	8.1	3.2	36.6
Vermont														
Burlington	593,348	191.0	73.1	116.0	8.3	5.2	11.9	10.5	5.6	6.2	15.5	8.5	3.9	38.9
Virginia														
Arlington	1,516,813	199.0	66.3	131.0	8.6	6.5	8.5	13.9	6.9	8.1	15.9	8.5	3.7	41.6
Charlottesville	431,219	209.3	76.4	130.6	9.5	4.7	11.9	11.0	5.5	6.8	16.3	11.2	3.6	61.7
Lynchburg	213,943	153.6	58.7	94.1	7.2	2.3	9.2	10.5	5.5	6.9	7.3	7.9	3.5	14.6
Newport News	470,475	178.3	62.0	115.0	8.8	5.5	8.9	13.7	5.9	7.2	12.6	7.1	3.4	24.7
Norfolk	1,124,582	192.2	62.1	128.8	10.0	5.4	11.6	13.7	5.8	7.3	11.5	8.2	4.7	40.9
Richmond	1,247,486	194.0	67.2	126.0	8.5	7.6	9.8	11.9	6.1	7.8	13.0	10.6	3.2	43.9
Roanoke	655,809	171.7	59.9	110.6	8.8	3.8	10.7	12.0	5.3	6.5	8.6	10.0	3.6	25.9
Winchester	294,525	158.0	54.3	102.7	8.4	4.4	10.9	10.8	6.0	8.1	7.5	6.9	4.3	12.7
Washington														
Everett	430,246	194.3	75.9	116.7	12.2	4.3	9.2	12.5	6.0	9.2	9.5	8.3	3.8	15.3
Olympia	264,075	184.4	71.9	111.9	11.8	2.7	8.5	11.7	6.1	8.5	7.5	8.9	4.0	19.8
Seattle	2,151,656	239.3	88.3	149.5	14.2	4.9	9.4	11.9	6.9	10.2	16.7	11.0	4.1	44.2
Spokane	1,083,197	181.3	70.4	109.3	9.5	4.3	7.7	10.1	5.8	8.7	9.7	8.3	2.9	12.9
Tacoma	589,030	201.8	67.9	131.7	14.1	4.9	8.1	10.6	6.3	10.3	12.5	10.4	3.2	34.9
Yakima	224,261	171.5	69.2	101.8	7.0	4.2	7.5	11.7	5.1	9.3	9.2	6.9	4.4	10.7
West Virginia														
Charleston	856,149	160.3	64.3	94.5	5.9	4.0	11.6	10.6	4.0	5.2	5.7	6.9	3.5	23.7
Huntington	349,438	155.9	54.4	99.9	5.9	5.1	10.9	11.0	4.4	5.2	8.4	8.0	3.6	31.8
Morgantown	376,117	173.4	65.1	107.5	7.4	3.7	9.0	9.2	4.8	6.3	7.5	9.9	3.9	54.3
Wisconsin														
Appleton	269,657	140.9	60.1	80.2	7.4	4.5	7.1	7.8	4.0	5.1	4.2	7.2	1.9	11.8
Green Bay	446,098	135.4	51.5	82.7	6.1	3.3	9.0	8.7	4.8	5.7	5.4	7.4	2.9	9.3
La Crosse	320,536	158.6	62.4	95.8	6.7	3.8	8.8	6.7	4.8	6.9	7.8	10.0	2.5	28.9
Madison	875,793	180.9	70.6	109.4	8.5	4.1	7.2	7.5	6.8	7.1	12.5	9.5	2.2	51.4
Marshfield	342,484	169.3	65.8	103.1	8.4	3.7	8.6	8.7	5.5	6.9	6.5	8.7	2.7	15.7
Milwaukee	2,326,759	182.8	61.1	120.8	11.7	5.2	8.6	10.9	5.8	7.9	12.0	10.0	3.0	41.0
Neenah	201,177	155.4	55.1	99.9	7.7	3.8	8.1	6.8	4.7	8.3	11.4	10.9	3.1	17.6
Wausau	167,971	173.9	68.9	104.4	8.2	4.8	9.4	9.3	5.6	7.7	7.7	11.1	3.1	12.1
Wyoming														
Casper	164,307	179.9	72.7	107.0	11.5	2.8	11.5	10.5	5.5	10.7	6.3	9.3	3.9	17.6
Large HMO														
HMO		125.2	56.2	69.0	7.8	2.3	4.5	8.8	4.5	4.5	2.9	8.7	2.8	
United States														
US	248,652,605	189.0	66.0	121.7	9.8	5.7	9.7	12.1	5.9	7.2	13.0	9.0	3.3	39.0

*All rates are age and sex adjusted and corrected for out of area use. See Part Nine, Section 5, for details. Physicians in residency training programs, regardless of specialty area, are grouped together. The count of primary care physicians added to the count of specialists does not equal the count of all physicians; the difference (about 1%) is attributable to the count of those in the All Physicians category whose specialty areas were identified as "unspecified."

Description of Variables for Table 3

Variable	Description	Price Adjustment	Figure List
Medicare Population, 1992 plus 1993	Approximately Double the actual Medicare Population, this is the denominator for calculating procedure rates from two years of Medicare Discharge Records		
Medicare Population, 1993	The Medicare Population in 1993 used as the denominator for Part B Rates.		
CABG Procedure Rate	Discharge Rate for CABG Surgery per 1000 Medicare Enrollees in HRRs		6.1, 6.3
PTCA Procedure Rate	Discharge Rate for PTCA per 1000 Medicare Enrollees in HRRs		6.2, 6.3
Part A Angiography Rate	Discharge Rate for Coronary Angiography per 1000 Medicare Enrollees in HRRs		6.3
Part B Prostate Biopsy Incidence Rate	Incidence of Prostate Biopsy per 1000 Medicare Male Enrollees from 1993 Part B Claims Records		6.7
Radical Prostatectomy Rate	Discharge Rate for Radical Prostatectomy per 1000 Medicare Male Enrollees in HRRs		6.8
Part B Mammography Incidence Rate	Incidence of Mammography per 1000 Medicare Female Enrollees from 1993 Part B Claims Records		6.4
Part A Percent Partial Mastectomies	Percent of Breast Sparing Surgery per 1000 Medicare Female Enrollees in HRRs		6.5
Back Surgery Rate	Discharge Rate for Back Surgery per 1000 Medicare Enrollees in HRRs		6.6
Hip Fracture Rate	Discharge Rate for Hip Fracture per 1000 Medicare Enrollees in HRRs		3.3, 3.7
Rate for High Variation Medical Conditions	Discharge Rate for High Variation Medical Conditions per 1000 Medicare Enrollees in HRRs		3.5, 3.7
Percent In-Hospital Medicare Deaths	Percent of Deaths among Medicare Enrollees that occurred in the Hospital for HRRs		3.6, 3.7
Rate for All Surgical Discharges	Surgical Discharge Rate per 1000 Medicare Enrollees in HRRs		3.4, 3.7
Medicare Mortality Rate	Mortality Rate per 1000 Medicare Enrollees in HRRs		3.8
TURP and BPH Rate	TURP and BPH Rate per 1000 Male Medicare Enrollees in HRRs		6.9

TABLE THREE

Selected Causes of Hospitalization, Diagnostic and Surgical Procedures, and Mortality Among Non-HMO Medicare Enrollees by Hospital Referral Region

(Rates are per 1,000 enrollee person-years and for 1992-93 except as indicated)*

Hospital Referral Region	Medicare Enrollees (1992 plus 1993)	Medicare Enrollees (1993 only)	CABG Surgery	PTCA	Coronary Angiography (1993)	Prostate Biopsy (1993)	Radical Prostatectomy	Mammography (1993)	Percentage Breast Sparing Surgery	Back Surgery	Hip Fracture	High Variation Medical Conditions	Percentage of Deaths Occurring in Hospitals	All Surgical Discharges	Medicare Mortality	TURP for BPH
Alabama																
Birmingham	533,325	267,273	7.7	7.7	30.9	23.1	2.53	219.3	8.1	3.6	8.8	243.8	47.0	109.6	53.6	13.4
Dothan	88,143	44,259	6.2	5.7	27.5	25.1	3.25	269.6	7.8	3.0	8.5	302.5	45.6	104.5	52.9	14.9
Huntsville	102,842	51,975	6.9	5.4	24.2	23.9	4.32	172.5	4.7	3.3	8.5	221.9	44.0	99.5	54.2	13.7
Mobile	162,260	81,643	7.7	6.0	25.7	21.0	2.41	216.0	11.4	2.8	8.8	238.2	43.6	111.5	52.3	9.5
Montgomery	97,212	48,516	4.9	9.2	26.5	25.7	3.63	217.3	12.0	4.4	8.3	226.4	44.9	105.8	51.8	10.8
Tuscaloosa	55,250	27,716	6.5	7.3	24.1	29.4	2.07	218.2	3.0	3.0	8.3	251.3	45.2	97.2	51.4	8.2
Alaska																
Anchorage	48,768	24,821	4.0	2.1	8.7	22.0	2.67	197.4	11.9	2.6	7.5	195.9	29.8	77.6	51.6	7.3
Arizona																
Mesa	160,951	57,254	4.3	4.1	14.0	16.1	3.67	239.5	7.3	3.1	7.4	139.3	30.2	90.6	46.8	11.8
Phoenix	458,829	191,774	4.3	4.8	13.2	18.3	3.18	218.4	9.9	2.5	8.3	153.1	28.8	92.2	52.2	13.2
Sun City	119,569	48,484	4.0	7.7	17.3	36.0	3.44	356.4	15.2	3.1	7.5	110.3	30.7	93.9	40.4	14.6
Tucson	227,366	86,986	3.7	5.3	16.3	25.1	3.00	193.7	10.7	4.0	8.0	148.8	27.9	89.3	51.1	13.7
Arkansas																
Fort Smith	88,576	44,277	4.9	3.5	15.8	25.6	2.78	160.3	4.3	2.2	8.5	235.5	44.0	94.9	55.0	19.0
Jonesboro	62,392	31,099	6.6	7.7	19.3	11.4	2.08	170.0	4.3	3.4	7.9	225.8	45.5	99.7	56.0	14.9
Little Rock	386,377	193,215	7.1	3.8	18.1	23.5	3.48	177.6	10.4	2.9	8.6	224.1	41.5	98.5	52.6	12.9
Springdale	91,691	46,032	4.4	4.8	16.5	25.4	1.68	212.2	8.3	2.2	8.3	178.9	35.6	86.4	50.2	13.7
Texarkana	70,646	35,094	7.3	1.8	15.2	21.7	0.96	167.2	5.9	3.4	8.0	234.5	44.8	94.8	54.5	13.1
California																
Orange Co.	445,745	148,733	4.6	5.4	13.4	26.8	4.52	247.2	17.8	3.2	7.4	161.7	34.4	90.3	51.5	10.6
Bakersfield	156,144	65,463	5.6	7.3	15.5	24.6	3.48	250.3	15.0	3.1	8.1	185.1	39.5	101.1	53.8	14.0
Chico	84,396	40,695	5.1	4.3	14.2	22.5	2.13	265.5	14.3	3.3	7.7	153.1	32.0	95.2	50.6	12.1
Contra Costa Co.	153,648	76,593	6.0	5.9	15.8	19.6	3.19	184.3	28.6	2.4	6.8	144.6	32.4	87.9	46.7	11.1
Fresno	175,695	87,954	4.3	4.1	11.5	24.6	4.95	254.1	16.7	2.5	6.7	133.1	31.2	83.0	47.6	13.4
Los Angeles	1,525,138	523,261	4.7	5.5	14.7	26.4	3.94	212.6	22.4	3.0	7.3	196.9	36.9	98.3	51.4	13.2
Modesto	142,217	71,424	6.0	6.3	15.4	18.8	2.84	250.4	16.5	3.3	7.2	169.6	38.9	96.6	48.1	14.5
Napa	77,378	38,599	6.6	11.6	24.2	21.2	2.42	232.6	19.2	2.7	8.0	156.2	29.7	110.9	49.7	13.1
Alameda Co.	261,720	128,493	4.0	7.4	11.7	14.3	2.14	184.2	23.4	2.7	7.0	154.6	32.3	86.4	48.0	11.6
Palm Spr/Rancho Mir	88,850	33,911	4.7	7.2	14.2	28.0	6.41	180.1	20.9	5.0	8.0	145.0	31.8	102.6	48.7	13.2
Redding	83,839	41,997	7.4	5.6	19.7	21.5	3.92	271.2	13.4	4.9	7.8	151.9	33.8	102.2	52.8	12.0
Sacramento	417,647	203,735	6.1	4.8	16.4	19.7	2.54	216.3	23.5	2.8	7.6	159.0	34.0	90.2	49.2	12.3
Salinas	65,409	32,877	4.8	10.7	17.6	24.7	1.66	201.2	16.7	3.5	6.2	136.2	27.7	94.2	47.1	10.5
San Bernardino	410,855	104,442	4.4	5.0	13.1	15.8	2.95	189.8	13.8	3.4	7.8	186.8	34.0	94.7	58.9	11.5
San Diego	580,299	185,903	4.3	4.8	13.4	28.6	3.93	211.0	22.7	4.1	7.5	148.9	29.5	92.4	52.5	11.7
San Francisco	303,017	137,196	4.1	3.6	10.8	17.3	2.64	184.5	28.4	2.5	6.7	151.8	32.1	79.1	47.4	9.2
San Jose	234,616	112,354	4.6	5.9	14.0	18.9	3.25	175.3	13.0	2.6	6.5	140.1	31.2	84.8	48.1	11.0
San Luis Obispo	58,520	29,144	4.4	4.1	11.5	12.8	3.64	300.1	18.9	4.2	6.4	131.8	28.4	86.5	45.6	13.9

Hospital Referral Region	Medicare Enrollees (1992 plus 1993)	Medicare Enrollees (1993 only)	CABG Surgery	PTCA	Coronary Angiography (1993)	Prostate Biopsy (1993)	Radical Prostatectomy	Mammography (1993)	Percentage Breast Sparing Surgery	Back Surgery	Hip Fracture	High Variation Medical Conditions	Percentage of Deaths Occurring in Hospitals	All Surgical Discharges	Medicare Mortality	TURP for BPH
San Mateo Co.	167,078	71,053	4.1	4.9	11.9	14.8	2.47	227.1	19.2	2.5	6.5	122.4	26.7	80.8	48.4	9.9
Santa Barbara	91,120	39,885	4.3	4.8	11.8	25.3	3.59	205.8	12.8	4.6	6.9	126.4	28.9	88.2	46.8	10.1
Santa Cruz	50,013	24,868	4.4	8.0	14.5	10.1	3.22	257.4	13.5	3.6	6.1	133.5	28.8	86.2	48.0	13.4
Santa Rosa	104,504	52,191	4.0	6.4	13.1	19.0	2.69	225.2	24.2	2.3	6.7	146.6	27.9	87.0	47.9	9.4
Stockton	85,687	42,941	5.9	12.8	23.0	17.3	1.68	262.0	20.1	2.2	6.9	162.0	38.4	97.6	50.2	9.7
Ventura	129,125	48,138	4.6	5.2	12.5	29.4	5.29	251.3	17.2	4.5	6.8	144.4	31.8	93.2	48.4	14.8
Colorado																
Boulder	34,094	14,906	3.1	3.0	8.3	13.8	6.70	214.6	13.3	4.4	8.8	145.3	27.4	88.7	46.8	13.4
Colorado Springs	117,417	56,562	4.8	4.6	14.0	14.4	1.73	186.7	10.2	3.0	8.3	150.9	30.7	85.1	46.7	12.7
Denver	380,137	163,270	3.1	4.5	13.5	23.2	3.65	193.8	17.2	3.2	8.0	161.0	29.5	90.1	50.7	13.2
Fort Collins	46,391	23,445	4.5	6.0	15.5	22.6	4.40	279.6	4.7	5.5	7.8	150.8	30.8	97.9	45.9	13.5
Grand Junction	57,417	29,020	2.1	3.8	8.9	22.1	3.13	145.5	14.8	3.5	7.3	139.7	24.2	87.7	45.5	7.1
Greeley	57,263	28,585	4.6	3.6	12.9	21.9	4.44	180.2	13.1	6.1	7.5	168.7	33.9	101.7	45.6	12.4
Pueblo	40,855	19,628	3.5	3.1	12.5	7.3	0.84	143.1	5.8	3.7	7.8	155.6	36.7	91.5	44.0	12.5
Connecticut																
Bridgeport	176,034	88,105	3.9	5.0	16.3	25.0	1.45	210.8	28.4	3.1	6.9	152.7	38.9	88.6	47.3	12.2
Hartford	375,616	188,277	5.7	3.7	14.1	25.3	1.81	243.9	28.1	2.2	7.1	153.1	36.9	91.8	48.0	10.4
New Haven	350,286	175,454	5.4	5.5	17.4	17.5	1.45	230.6	21.8	2.0	6.8	155.2	35.1	90.4	48.7	9.4
Delaware																
Wilmington	146,322	73,666	4.6	5.6	17.4	26.5	2.06	252.9	13.4	2.7	7.4	187.5	39.1	102.2	55.0	16.5
District of Columbia																
Washington	424,100	212,972	4.7	4.9	14.4	32.9	2.67	240.9	17.5	2.9	7.2	196.7	42.0	97.2	49.5	13.8
Florida																
Bradenton	97,119	48,677	6.2	3.9	17.2	26.6	2.29	280.9	19.9	3.9	7.5	132.4	36.7	89.6	45.0	11.1
Clearwater	217,939	96,789	5.0	5.2	17.4	31.0	4.10	326.9	28.3	4.0	7.9	165.7	37.4	100.3	45.3	14.0
Fort Lauderdale	842,301	333,215	6.3	6.4	17.2	38.1	2.49	341.7	27.0	2.9	7.8	162.7	35.9	95.2	43.7	12.9
Fort Myers	310,935	157,591	5.4	5.5	17.4	37.5	4.55	283.1	14.1	5.5	7.1	157.3	35.5	99.1	42.1	10.7
Gainesville	105,665	53,306	5.8	3.8	15.9	16.3	2.15	248.8	16.4	3.2	8.0	191.3	32.9	91.8	53.0	15.9
Hudson	192,235	86,583	7.2	5.0	17.7	47.1	3.23	302.1	10.3	4.5	7.4	189.4	41.3	104.8	46.8	17.5
Jacksonville	255,066	128,785	6.6	5.7	21.9	35.0	2.38	226.8	12.4	2.7	8.2	206.6	38.2	99.1	53.2	10.6
Lakeland	85,927	41,935	5.2	7.6	19.5	43.3	2.83	258.4	12.2	3.4	8.4	149.9	35.9	88.0	48.3	12.2
Miami	651,143	236,134	4.9	4.8	14.3	34.2	2.21	242.0	19.5	1.4	8.1	198.8	42.2	91.1	47.4	11.7
Ocala	159,246	81,014	6.4	5.2	16.3	47.2	3.66	279.0	14.0	3.3	6.9	139.9	33.1	93.0	45.0	11.7
Orlando	735,288	346,135	5.7	6.5	18.0	40.4	3.98	258.2	11.3	2.8	7.6	166.1	36.8	97.5	47.3	13.3
Ormond Beach	125,122	45,451	4.5	5.7	13.3	35.5	5.73	216.8	11.7	2.7	8.1	139.8	37.9	98.1	49.4	18.1
Panama City	41,831	21,241	4.8	5.4	23.3	24.0	1.60	241.2	3.8	2.4	8.2	231.0	44.5	100.1	54.5	14.6
Pensacola	141,193	71,683	5.7	4.7	18.7	21.9	3.64	204.0	11.2	3.9	8.1	214.7	42.1	97.4	51.9	8.9
Sarasota	186,748	93,972	6.5	5.8	17.9	32.3	5.76	337.9	9.9	3.6	7.9	136.3	33.0	99.6	42.0	13.6
St Petersburg	172,097	72,798	4.7	3.7	15.2	32.5	4.64	266.0	17.9	3.9	8.7	174.5	40.6	109.0	50.5	13.8
Tallahassee	143,433	71,944	4.8	3.1	14.3	33.2	2.51	205.2	6.7	3.2	8.3	210.4	39.2	95.8	53.5	18.3
Tampa	229,592	94,672	5.5	5.0	16.7	28.6	2.20	214.3	14.7	3.3	8.0	168.8	38.7	96.1	50.8	14.0
Georgia																
Albany	44,002	22,092	4.7	2.4	13.0	24.0	2.65	232.0	14.1	2.2	8.5	196.5	43.8	101.6	52.2	17.0
Atlanta	681,050	343,564	5.3	6.4	19.7	32.1	3.20	199.7	14.2	2.4	8.8	222.9	41.4	99.5	53.1	11.9
Augusta	121,770	61,150	5.5	9.9	21.7	15.8	1.37	203.6	6.9	2.7	8.0	213.3	41.9	93.5	57.0	6.5
Columbus	66,225	33,178	5.6	5.1	14.9	18.8	2.22	166.4	7.2	2.2	8.8	190.6	41.8	99.3	55.9	19.6

Hospital Referral Region	Medicare Enrollees (1992 plus 1993)	Medicare Enrollees (1993 only)	CABG Surgery	PTCA	Coronary Angiography (1993)	Prostate Biopsy (1993)	Radical Prostatectomy	Mammography (1993)	Percentage Breast Sparing Surgery	Back Surgery	Hip Fracture	High Variation Medical Conditions	Percentage of Deaths Occurring in Hospitals	All Surgical Discharges	Medicare Mortality	TURP for BPH
Macon	144,152	72,254	6.5	5.1	22.6	21.9	2.03	196.3	11.6	2.9	8.6	240.0	43.9	104.6	55.9	14.3
Rome	60,002	30,054	8.1	8.3	27.4	45.5	1.26	159.3	7.4	2.6	9.4	243.0	41.2	98.9	59.5	12.1
Savannah	136,605	68,864	6.3	5.2	19.2	31.2	2.79	231.5	13.8	4.4	7.8	227.8	44.0	99.4	51.8	10.1
Hawaii																
Honolulu	249,501	91,283	3.4	3.7	8.2	21.1	1.88	176.4	21.3	1.4	5.2	122.5	37.7	63.3	43.1	8.0
Idaho																
Boise	136,451	68,514	4.2	4.2	11.5	22.5	2.77	135.5	12.6	4.8	6.7	134.0	26.8	88.9	47.6	11.2
Idaho Falls	31,980	16,155	4.1	2.9	11.2	11.1	3.71	154.5	5.3	3.7	6.6	131.9	26.9	81.1	48.7	14.6
Illinois																
Aurora	33,092	16,567	5.3	4.1	17.1	12.3	1.20	142.7	23.3	2.8	7.6	174.0	36.4	96.2	51.4	12.8
Blue Island	208,834	96,480	6.2	5.1	19.8	25.4	2.88	157.3	18.0	2.4	7.3	227.7	37.4	101.3	57.2	13.6
Chicago	555,335	252,551	5.4	5.0	18.5	17.0	1.27	157.7	18.3	1.7	6.9	234.7	40.4	96.4	53.9	14.7
Elgin	83,405	40,361	4.7	5.5	16.0	21.0	1.78	128.0	14.5	3.4	7.5	194.0	35.6	95.1	54.3	14.0
Evanston	231,368	108,566	5.7	6.1	16.6	24.4	2.39	246.6	33.0	2.6	7.1	190.7	35.0	95.0	47.1	13.2
Hinsdale	61,934	30,199	7.5	5.4	20.0	32.5	3.52	199.6	22.0	3.0	7.0	174.0	32.2	93.9	50.3	10.3
Joliet	95,883	47,952	8.5	4.8	20.7	25.7	2.85	196.6	13.3	2.3	6.7	249.0	44.3	102.5	54.3	12.4
Melrose Park	289,360	134,345	6.7	5.0	19.9	17.0	1.66	175.3	19.3	2.4	6.9	190.4	35.0	94.8	52.4	13.7
Peoria	189,075	94,601	5.5	5.3	17.9	33.5	2.92	228.0	10.6	1.9	7.7	183.1	37.1	93.6	49.4	12.3
Rockford	169,883	85,221	4.2	6.1	16.5	20.7	3.07	176.6	11.8	2.0	7.5	179.5	34.8	90.9	48.7	11.3
Springfield	259,570	129,574	5.9	5.0	19.5	20.2	2.13	169.8	13.2	3.2	7.7	221.9	37.7	100.3	49.9	13.7
Urbana	112,448	56,222	5.1	4.1	14.5	21.7	2.00	241.8	16.8	2.6	7.4	190.9	35.1	91.0	52.1	13.8
Bloomington	37,816	18,958	7.8	2.9	19.1	30.1	2.09	232.3	3.0	2.9	7.7	191.3	34.4	94.2	50.8	11.7
Indiana																
Evansville	197,282	98,732	5.7	5.0	17.5	19.9	2.13	166.4	15.1	3.2	8.1	233.9	37.2	90.7	54.0	11.7
Fort Wayne	194,099	97,436	4.9	5.8	16.4	13.9	1.92	154.7	10.0	3.3	7.5	160.7	32.4	88.0	51.4	9.9
Gary	112,583	56,602	7.1	6.4	22.1	28.0	1.92	133.3	7.3	3.4	6.8	233.5	39.7	106.6	56.6	18.9
Indianapolis	572,482	285,128	4.9	6.6	16.7	18.5	2.24	179.6	18.5	2.5	8.2	207.7	38.8	95.4	54.3	12.3
Lafayette	45,501	22,767	5.7	7.3	20.4	6.6	2.61	106.8	9.1	2.9	7.4	160.8	32.6	87.9	52.8	11.8
Muncie	45,674	22,925	4.2	5.9	12.6	24.4	2.77	178.1	12.8	2.9	8.7	200.9	38.0	92.6	54.6	13.0
Munster	83,001	40,981	6.3	11.1	27.4	20.1	2.59	153.2	10.4	2.3	6.5	231.3	44.1	110.9	56.4	17.6
South Bend	165,290	83,059	5.8	3.1	13.3	18.1	1.72	143.9	7.7	2.4	7.2	158.0	32.6	87.6	51.5	10.9
Terre Haute	55,263	27,493	5.4	8.6	20.2	15.5	2.48	123.0	11.2	3.0	8.1	190.9	38.6	93.7	56.4	9.0
Iowa																
Cedar Rapids	70,096	35,134	6.8	3.6	17.1	32.6	3.53	172.5	8.1	3.1	7.7	159.5	35.7	99.3	46.0	11.2
Davenport	138,262	69,196	5.2	4.8	14.8	23.2	3.56	172.9	9.8	2.5	8.0	187.8	38.3	94.2	51.7	8.7
Des Moines	279,629	139,263	5.0	8.5	20.2	20.8	2.37	201.0	8.0	2.4	7.9	190.3	36.2	100.1	47.1	11.1
Dubuque	42,821	21,508	3.6	5.7	12.8	7.2	2.42	148.0	7.4	3.4	7.6	174.9	31.0	94.1	50.6	12.9
Iowa City	84,837	42,355	6.0	3.9	15.1	13.2	2.05	187.0	12.1	1.9	7.5	180.9	34.2	89.7	48.6	8.6
Mason City	54,183	27,052	6.6	5.1	17.4	7.5	2.05	206.1	6.3	4.1	7.4	154.2	29.2	97.6	45.3	14.9
Sioux City	80,675	40,261	3.5	5.4	14.2	22.4	2.08	200.4	7.0	2.8	7.8	165.5	31.8	97.9	46.6	15.5
Waterloo	64,146	32,055	4.5	3.0	11.4	26.4	4.48	180.6	12.4	2.4	7.9	175.7	33.1	93.4	48.7	11.0
Kansas																
Topeka	110,532	55,327	4.5	6.1	15.8	35.4	4.27	192.6	9.6	1.8	8.2	158.1	32.9	95.8	46.7	18.4
Wichita	352,720	173,960	5.9	6.2	19.8	25.8	3.18	199.1	11.4	3.0	8.3	203.6	37.3	100.9	46.7	16.5
Kentucky																
Covington	72,402	36,323	6.7	4.1	19.5	21.6	2.46	139.9	9.1	2.5	8.5	234.6	38.7	89.5	57.7	9.7

Hospital Referral Region	Medicare Enrollees (1992 plus 1993)	Medicare Enrollees (1993 only)	CABG Surgery	PTCA	Coronary Angiography (1993)	Prostate Biopsy (1993)	Radical Prostatectomy	Mammography (1993)	Percentage Breast Sparing Surgery	Back Surgery	Hip Fracture	High Variation Medical Conditions	Percentage of Deaths Occurring in Hospitals	All Surgical Discharges	Medicare Mortality	TURP for BPH
Lexington	297,538	149,367	5.5	2.8	13.8	16.6	1.91	161.7	7.0	1.6	8.3	263.1	43.1	80.3	56.8	12.9
Louisville	371,995	184,422	6.1	4.0	17.1	18.7	1.47	184.1	10.5	2.5	8.1	240.5	41.7	93.8	55.0	12.5
Owensboro	35,548	17,827	6.6	5.0	18.7	20.1	3.17	214.5	9.2	3.9	7.6	246.8	44.2	101.2	55.9	23.7
Paducah	113,578	56,798	6.3	3.9	23.3	17.7	2.45	223.5	19.7	3.0	8.8	257.6	45.1	102.0	51.9	12.7
Louisiana																
Alexandria	68,740	33,956	4.7	9.9	26.8	22.1	1.14	119.7	12.1	2.8	7.3	273.9	47.1	100.3	55.2	9.9
Baton Rouge	141,214	70,303	5.3	6.3	16.0	42.7	4.20	178.1	11.2	2.3	8.3	216.5	42.8	93.7	53.7	12.9
Houma	44,643	22,428	7.4	10.2	37.5	48.7	3.37	168.8	8.4	3.1	7.6	248.8	45.5	122.0	53.3	12.9
Lafayette	114,996	57,451	5.8	9.2	23.3	14.5	0.64	156.4	4.5	2.3	6.2	230.2	42.0	102.0	51.9	14.4
Lake Charles	50,898	25,554	4.8	7.2	21.2	22.6	1.80	173.5	10.2	3.1	7.0	278.4	49.2	102.0	54.3	12.0
Metairie	90,629	45,778	6.6	7.0	23.1	33.9	3.00	158.3	22.0	2.5	8.1	236.6	42.4	105.8	53.8	12.2
Monroe	69,164	33,888	5.6	3.9	17.7	23.8	1.90	159.9	11.1	3.8	8.2	323.8	45.5	102.3	52.9	17.9
New Orleans	183,269	91,028	6.4	7.5	22.4	18.4	2.13	145.6	15.1	2.2	7.6	221.7	39.2	106.1	54.2	11.1
Shreveport	169,892	83,987	4.8	5.9	20.0	24.4	2.15	145.0	6.1	3.5	7.9	219.4	42.5	95.5	51.0	16.3
Slidell	30,100	15,398	7.1	4.7	24.9	11.8	2.72	192.3	14.9	3.6	8.4	286.7	43.5	110.1	58.3	10.5
Maine																
Bangor	108,853	54,720	4.5	3.1	13.8	17.6	1.41	234.1	17.3	1.9	6.7	220.9	41.6	92.0	52.2	13.7
Portland	254,192	127,579	4.6	4.0	14.9	18.8	1.58	246.9	22.1	2.4	6.9	189.7	39.6	91.9	50.6	11.5
Maryland																
Baltimore	548,831	274,625	5.6	5.2	16.2	33.2	3.18	256.3	17.0	3.4	7.5	230.8	40.9	113.5	53.5	15.9
Salisbury	101,048	51,104	4.5	7.5	21.7	26.7	1.27	234.8	19.4	2.3	6.6	205.9	37.0	101.0	53.9	13.0
Takoma Park	128,043	64,654	4.6	7.1	17.7	27.9	1.83	238.3	10.4	2.8	7.3	179.5	41.5	97.8	48.6	11.8
Massachusetts																
Boston	1,177,153	578,227	4.6	3.6	13.5	20.0	2.17	251.4	31.7	1.9	7.2	220.9	41.4	95.9	49.1	14.3
Springfield	206,398	102,782	3.8	2.8	9.5	20.9	1.44	189.2	25.5	2.0	7.0	177.8	39.1	85.0	50.7	9.9
Worcester	191,634	78,247	4.3	2.9	10.5	18.8	1.69	223.3	26.8	2.0	7.2	221.8	41.9	94.4	52.5	15.1
Michigan																
Ann Arbor	255,856	128,729	5.5	5.6	15.5	27.9	2.64	300.3	25.8	2.4	6.9	182.2	35.9	94.0	52.2	12.6
Dearborn	144,988	72,348	6.8	5.7	15.3	43.5	2.97	273.3	13.8	1.7	6.3	189.7	43.4	94.6	54.5	12.0
Detroit	471,035	233,448	5.9	5.7	15.8	37.5	2.76	296.1	18.5	2.1	6.7	198.9	41.4	95.1	54.8	13.4
Flint	112,112	56,620	6.8	5.8	14.3	34.3	4.19	344.6	19.1	2.4	6.8	209.2	44.4	105.9	56.5	15.9
Grand Rapids	220,365	110,852	4.4	3.3	10.7	29.6	3.42	301.7	17.9	4.4	7.3	137.4	28.4	87.6	48.3	14.4
Kalamazoo	152,079	76,422	5.7	9.6	15.5	29.1	4.04	238.3	15.5	3.6	7.2	148.8	31.6	100.0	52.0	12.2
Lansing	130,755	62,071	6.1	4.5	14.0	22.4	3.98	347.0	22.4	3.3	7.1	176.0	35.8	99.7	51.9	12.0
Marquette	65,474	32,731	5.8	4.1	12.2	18.8	2.97	274.2	9.1	2.4	7.0	176.8	32.9	91.6	50.4	11.9
Muskegon	67,929	34,125	4.5	3.3	9.7	26.8	4.05	336.5	11.0	3.4	7.3	133.0	30.5	92.5	51.2	12.4
Petoskey	48,593	24,459	5.6	4.9	13.2	15.1	2.76	295.7	20.7	3.3	6.2	164.6	30.3	93.5	50.2	11.7
Pontiac	67,263	34,300	5.4	5.1	16.4	45.7	3.02	304.9	23.7	3.8	7.5	213.0	38.1	95.0	57.0	13.2
Royal Oak	159,500	80,077	5.9	6.8	17.0	46.6	3.32	355.6	25.2	2.7	6.9	173.1	39.7	93.7	48.3	14.0
Saginaw	185,287	93,134	7.2	7.9	17.4	32.5	3.44	303.5	11.3	3.7	6.0	194.6	35.5	106.3	50.6	15.3
St Joseph	38,816	19,488	5.6	9.2	19.6	39.4	3.69	334.9	8.9	3.4	6.3	154.7	37.6	92.5	51.6	7.3
Traverse City	60,606	30,614	7.0	6.2	16.5	23.7	1.77	319.8	14.8	3.8	7.0	179.7	32.7	102.5	48.5	11.9
Minnesota																
Duluth	110,860	55,265	3.8	4.0	11.9	19.3	1.53	164.4	5.0	2.4	6.8	173.7	34.8	93.2	47.7	19.4
Minneapolis	630,496	278,212	4.4	4.5	13.9	16.5	3.31	159.9	13.2	2.6	7.1	169.1	29.2	91.5	46.3	12.1
Rochester	110,641	55,172	4.3	5.0	15.5	15.3	3.53	183.4	14.5	1.9	7.2	172.1	30.4	90.4	45.1	11.6

Hospital Referral Region	Medicare Enrollees (1992 plus 1993)	Medicare Enrollees (1993 only)	CABG Surgery	PTCA	Coronary Angiography (1993)	Prostate Biopsy (1993)	Radical Prostatectomy	Mammography (1993)	Percentage Breast Sparing Surgery	Back Surgery	Hip Fracture	High Variation Medical Conditions	Percentage of Deaths Occurring in Hospitals	All Surgical Discharges	Medicare Mortality	TURP for BPH
St Cloud	50,192	25,133	4.3	3.9	11.8	17.2	3.25	219.1	15.9	3.0	6.5	172.3	28.0	85.2	44.2	11.8
St Paul	185,089	71,704	4.2	4.3	11.8	20.8	4.95	188.1	13.0	2.6	7.4	183.5	27.1	94.3	48.4	12.2
Mississippi																
Gulfport	36,690	18,555	4.9	4.7	18.2	12.7	2.25	206.2	3.4	2.5	7.9	280.6	46.2	109.4	59.0	12.3
Hattiesburg	63,460	31,739	4.2	4.1	17.7	33.6	5.51	190.2	8.9	2.6	8.2	284.9	50.2	107.4	54.9	14.6
Jackson	240,661	119,625	4.2	2.7	12.4	26.5	4.12	189.7	9.3	2.6	8.1	250.1	45.5	88.4	51.9	13.4
Meridian	53,603	26,687	4.3	2.6	13.3	33.0	2.85	235.4	11.5	1.7	7.7	290.6	48.9	86.9	50.2	10.8
Oxford	34,523	17,195	5.8	4.5	21.4	21.0	1.26	114.9	5.0	3.5	8.8	278.5	49.2	101.0	49.2	14.9
Tupelo	89,043	44,485	4.6	2.4	15.3	22.3	1.58	155.8	2.8	2.9	8.2	249.2	48.6	88.2	51.3	11.0
Missouri																
Cape Girardeau	77,388	38,572	5.7	6.5	17.4	28.9	2.03	121.4	5.4	3.3	7.8	167.1	39.3	87.9	52.8	13.4
Columbia	178,080	88,769	6.9	7.3	20.3	30.2	3.50	127.9	8.0	3.3	7.7	180.4	34.9	100.2	50.0	14.1
Joplin	105,302	52,556	5.1	6.3	19.6	19.1	2.59	161.5	4.9	2.6	8.5	235.5	38.3	101.6	53.5	17.3
Kansas City	507,563	241,129	5.1	6.7	18.6	26.4	4.80	179.7	13.5	2.6	8.7	190.6	34.7	97.2	51.8	13.9
Springfield	211,518	106,164	5.3	9.0	23.8	33.3	3.88	184.3	6.8	2.9	8.4	178.8	33.0	97.6	50.5	18.3
St Louis	837,617	418,988	6.1	5.2	18.0	28.3	4.81	165.8	13.8	2.8	8.1	202.1	37.7	99.5	52.6	12.4
Montana																
Billings	120,822	60,821	5.4	4.1	13.0	34.2	5.74	189.7	16.9	3.8	8.0	193.5	29.9	94.5	48.2	8.5
Great Falls	39,696	19,886	4.4	5.6	15.6	28.2	3.57	209.4	15.5	2.2	7.6	230.3	33.9	91.3	48.0	9.5
Missoula	82,422	41,374	4.1	9.4	18.4	29.5	3.29	169.1	9.6	3.0	7.8	195.0	29.3	98.9	49.7	14.9
Nebraska																
Lincoln	158,565	79,126	4.9	3.2	11.2	17.2	2.98	176.7	12.3	2.3	7.3	133.9	30.3	89.0	46.3	12.9
Omaha	308,292	151,270	5.0	5.1	15.6	25.9	3.68	168.2	9.9	3.1	7.9	165.9	34.3	95.6	48.7	13.7
Nevada																
Las Vegas	207,303	86,110	5.4	5.8	15.9	40.4	2.74	171.5	10.6	2.8	7.7	159.1	40.4	95.9	57.9	12.5
Reno	118,820	59,800	4.0	4.0	12.5	21.7	3.18	162.2	17.6	2.4	7.9	149.6	31.6	80.7	52.4	7.5
New Hampshire																
Lebanon	106,343	53,424	3.3	2.0	8.2	20.8	1.68	219.9	14.9	2.3	6.9	163.8	32.7	78.7	49.7	11.6
Manchester	164,646	82,822	5.2	3.5	15.3	18.7	1.82	192.6	21.9	2.6	7.2	159.7	34.6	85.7	50.1	10.6
New Jersey																
Camden	711,959	357,129	5.1	3.9	17.7	29.4	1.35	206.8	21.7	1.7	7.1	219.3	50.8	100.4	52.2	13.1
Hackensack	316,870	158,231	4.7	3.9	14.1	28.2	1.92	164.2	30.9	1.5	6.9	187.6	49.8	99.1	48.2	17.4
Morristown	204,182	102,808	4.3	3.8	15.0	39.8	3.31	203.5	23.8	1.8	7.4	189.1	44.2	94.8	49.0	14.7
New Brunswick	190,802	96,187	4.7	5.1	19.4	31.4	2.57	186.6	31.6	2.2	7.0	204.7	50.3	98.2	52.1	13.0
Newark	360,757	179,074	4.6	4.7	18.9	27.1	1.58	161.8	21.4	1.2	6.8	226.1	53.5	100.8	52.7	17.9
Paterson	82,760	41,470	4.5	4.0	15.9	31.7	1.54	167.6	37.8	1.5	6.7	197.9	48.3	96.0	53.1	16.0
Ridgewood	87,371	43,825	5.0	3.4	12.5	37.0	2.76	202.9	34.8	1.6	7.1	185.1	43.6	90.5	49.8	11.9
New Mexico																
Albuquerque	264,319	117,763	2.7	2.9	10.4	24.9	3.48	142.2	15.7	2.5	8.0	160.2	29.3	80.2	46.0	10.3
New York																
Albany	480,393	240,305	5.3	2.4	10.2	23.6	1.76	208.6	28.4	1.8	7.3	186.4	42.3	87.9	51.5	12.5
Binghamton	110,194	55,190	4.5	3.2	13.3	30.6	1.76	259.2	22.9	2.4	7.0	198.8	40.2	87.4	50.4	11.2
Bronx	231,446	109,294	3.5	2.6	11.5	21.5	1.36	164.2	31.5	1.1	6.7	203.2	50.6	92.0	50.8	14.2
Buffalo	430,720	210,491	5.0	1.6	12.3	27.1	1.83	243.0	16.9	1.7	6.8	181.8	48.7	88.0	53.6	12.5
Elmira	111,156	55,460	5.2	3.6	14.5	35.6	1.84	283.0	23.4	1.5	7.0	198.7	41.4	85.5	52.0	11.2
East Long Island	1,075,989	508,296	4.7	3.7	13.3	26.9	1.48	213.8	30.4	1.2	6.8	181.9	52.7	90.2	50.0	12.9

Hospital Referral Region	Medicare Enrollees (1992 plus 1993)	Medicare Enrollees (1993 only)	CABG Surgery	PTCA	Coronary Angiography (1993)	Prostate Biopsy (1993)	Radical Prostatectomy	Mammography (1993)	Percentage Breast Sparing Surgery	Back Surgery	Hip Fracture	High Variation Medical Conditions	Percentage of Deaths Occurring in Hospitals	All Surgical Discharges	Medicare Mortality	TURP for BPH
New York	1,012,093	475,687	4.4	2.8	12.3	27.2	1.15	213.8	29.3	1.2	6.8	178.1	51.8	90.8	47.7	12.8
Rochester	311,540	148,825	4.8	2.5	12.2	17.9	1.97	264.8	25.5	2.1	7.3	174.3	40.4	90.8	51.6	12.2
Syracuse	267,579	134,058	4.0	2.8	10.8	20.5	2.28	289.1	18.1	1.5	6.8	175.1	40.8	86.9	51.9	10.4
White Plains	265,574	131,886	3.8	2.5	10.0	25.2	2.32	208.5	30.1	1.7	6.9	196.3	46.0	92.1	47.2	13.9
North Carolina																
Asheville	176,098	88,828	3.9	2.4	9.9	22.5	4.24	200.5	8.5	3.4	8.3	166.7	35.9	84.5	48.6	12.2
Charlotte	372,100	187,765	4.9	4.6	17.6	30.7	3.39	156.3	10.9	3.0	9.3	157.9	40.1	87.1	53.5	10.9
Durham	280,019	141,273	5.7	4.5	18.6	21.9	3.74	210.0	12.3	2.7	8.3	163.1	39.0	86.5	52.5	12.2
Greensboro	121,709	61,470	5.5	6.9	19.8	21.5	3.18	189.4	8.5	3.4	8.9	164.4	36.3	94.1	52.7	12.8
Greenville	159,535	80,765	6.2	4.7	15.8	16.8	2.06	196.5	9.4	2.9	8.5	182.9	40.8	91.2	54.9	8.5
Hickory	58,787	29,765	5.5	4.2	15.8	26.9	3.54	163.3	3.4	3.2	8.7	164.7	38.9	88.4	52.0	9.0
Raleigh	253,253	128,251	5.3	4.3	14.7	21.9	2.86	187.2	9.5	3.6	8.3	177.1	43.0	91.3	54.3	10.5
Wilmington	77,736	39,504	5.5	3.9	13.3	24.6	2.74	183.4	8.2	2.9	8.4	186.0	40.4	94.0	55.0	9.5
Winston-Salem	237,676	119,943	5.5	4.5	17.2	25.6	3.55	176.9	5.9	2.9	8.7	188.8	43.3	95.1	52.8	14.1
North Dakota																
Bismarck	61,250	30,726	6.0	3.9	13.6	25.8	3.91	255.6	6.2	4.1	6.4	218.4	34.1	99.9	44.6	13.3
Fargo Moorhead -Mn	144,770	72,408	4.9	4.1	12.3	24.2	2.77	213.6	4.5	2.4	7.0	170.4	33.8	93.4	44.9	12.6
Grand Forks	49,928	24,851	5.6	4.4	16.3	21.4	1.83	152.6	6.1	2.3	7.3	179.0	30.5	86.4	48.3	11.6
Minot	39,390	19,663	6.6	5.4	15.2	36.2	7.11	260.4	6.5	2.5	7.8	183.5	31.5	98.9	41.9	19.7
Ohio																
Akron	178,666	88,492	6.4	5.5	19.2	21.5	1.78	210.3	11.5	3.0	7.8	215.6	43.0	98.4	54.0	10.1
Canton	169,709	85,218	5.3	3.5	13.8	16.8	1.52	194.2	10.8	2.7	7.6	172.6	35.0	87.0	52.4	11.3
Cincinnati	364,410	182,646	5.8	5.4	17.7	21.4	2.37	174.1	14.9	2.9	8.0	198.6	35.1	94.7	54.1	14.2
Cleveland	601,249	287,654	5.9	4.0	15.5	23.0	2.16	213.1	23.0	2.8	7.1	203.6	38.3	100.3	52.2	12.3
Columbus	589,377	296,162	4.7	5.9	18.4	24.0	2.59	180.9	11.6	2.1	7.9	202.1	36.3	97.2	54.8	13.6
Dayton	279,090	140,131	6.8	6.2	20.1	18.5	2.19	184.5	12.8	3.1	7.9	188.7	33.4	99.4	53.2	11.2
Elyria	58,453	29,207	5.5	9.1	21.9	29.4	1.58	209.5	48.0	2.7	6.8	220.8	34.3	114.0	53.2	13.5
Kettering	90,751	45,859	6.3	4.6	17.7	24.7	3.68	183.1	15.1	2.3	8.3	166.7	34.3	95.6	51.1	12.6
Toledo	248,902	124,817	4.3	4.4	13.6	34.9	2.32	188.7	13.4	3.4	7.8	209.3	37.0	105.3	53.7	13.5
Youngstown	230,392	115,687	5.5	4.1	15.2	30.3	2.29	242.6	20.3	2.5	7.1	226.1	41.1	103.9	53.4	17.0
Oklahoma																
Lawton	48,282	24,123	5.9	4.4	13.5	20.8	1.64	145.3	14.3	3.3	8.6	178.4	40.3	88.2	50.8	9.9
Oklahoma City	413,680	204,818	5.6	6.0	18.5	28.3	4.70	131.2	11.7	3.2	8.6	204.0	43.8	102.7	52.4	15.5
Tulsa	302,808	146,680	4.5	5.5	15.9	22.7	2.49	182.7	8.1	3.3	8.9	182.4	39.1	90.4	52.6	12.4
Oregon																
Bend	37,767	18,970	4.3	6.2	13.4	29.2	4.57	178.6	9.6	6.1	8.1	115.5	22.8	107.3	46.2	19.5
Eugene	175,298	84,848	4.0	3.9	10.5	24.8	4.51	203.6	18.9	5.2	7.7	135.2	24.6	90.6	49.6	14.0
Medford	123,096	61,774	4.3	2.4	9.9	15.0	2.52	207.2	8.0	4.1	7.0	126.1	24.5	82.6	48.2	11.2
Portland	492,638	168,475	4.2	3.8	10.5	20.7	4.44	181.1	17.1	4.4	7.4	135.8	22.8	84.9	55.2	11.5
Salem	66,808	28,785	4.4	4.0	10.2	20.7	3.72	164.1	15.3	4.1	7.3	108.1	29.0	82.3	50.3	9.2
Pennsylvania																
Allentown	307,630	153,538	5.3	4.6	19.0	33.6	1.79	225.6	18.7	2.1	6.9	212.6	43.1	107.7	51.2	16.6
Altoona	95,138	47,695	6.1	2.5	13.8	20.1	0.88	188.3	20.4	2.1	7.3	219.1	40.9	92.1	53.6	15.3
Danville	156,618	78,692	4.7	2.8	13.2	24.2	2.05	241.9	17.8	2.8	7.0	208.1	38.8	96.9	52.5	14.6
Erie	224,883	112,798	4.6	4.2	13.8	22.6	2.20	217.3	19.8	2.3	7.6	220.1	39.1	94.2	52.6	13.2
Harrisburg	247,967	124,918	5.3	4.9	16.8	34.9	3.44	259.0	15.6	2.6	7.4	180.7	38.2	95.8	51.6	10.9

Hospital Referral Region	Medicare Enrollees (1992 plus 1993)	Medicare Enrollees (1993 only)	CABG Surgery	PTCA	Coronary Angiography (1993)	Prostate Biopsy (1993)	Radical Prostatectomy	Mammography (1993)	Percentage Breast Sparing Surgery	Back Surgery	Hip Fracture	High Variation Medical Conditions	Percentage of Deaths Occurring in Hospitals	All Surgical Discharges	Medicare Mortality	TURP for BPH
Johnstown	88,606	44,399	6.0	5.5	20.8	25.7	1.82	169.2	32.2	2.6	6.7	273.5	43.4	105.4	52.3	13.3
Lancaster	137,147	69,132	6.0	5.9	23.4	33.5	4.44	207.5	16.4	4.3	7.0	168.4	30.4	100.0	47.7	12.5
Philadelphia	1,088,052	522,192	5.4	4.3	18.5	24.0	1.99	222.3	30.6	2.0	7.5	227.1	45.0	107.0	52.7	14.6
Pittsburgh	1,046,066	523,354	5.6	5.8	20.5	26.6	2.21	198.0	31.7	2.6	7.3	260.7	43.5	107.3	54.1	13.2
Reading	170,594	85,239	5.5	5.0	21.2	23.4	1.79	176.6	15.5	3.0	6.7	187.9	41.3	98.2	52.8	12.9
Sayre	55,790	28,008	4.0	3.0	14.6	20.7	0.90	210.3	14.1	2.1	7.2	215.2	40.0	92.0	50.6	9.7
Scranton	116,239	58,229	4.9	3.5	14.4	25.0	1.04	169.3	18.4	2.3	7.3	213.2	46.0	96.0	54.9	11.6
Wilkes-Barre	99,035	49,540	5.4	2.2	14.5	24.2	1.17	158.6	16.3	1.8	6.4	227.9	44.1	95.8	55.1	12.4
York	95,174	47,991	4.7	2.3	10.6	25.4	1.45	215.2	11.1	1.9	7.1	150.8	32.7	92.4	48.9	15.0
Rhode Island																
Providence	323,129	152,455	4.3	3.2	11.5	20.2	1.21	189.6	22.4	1.6	7.0	189.1	37.6	89.9	50.6	12.6
South Carolina																
Charleston	149,532	76,139	4.8	5.5	17.3	29.2	3.75	226.4	7.8	3.4	7.4	180.1	42.3	97.9	51.6	15.4
Columbia	215,258	108,229	5.3	4.9	17.6	21.8	2.14	141.8	6.8	2.2	7.8	160.1	40.6	85.7	52.8	10.1
Florence	76,879	38,625	5.1	7.3	20.4	31.1	0.89	234.4	8.3	2.7	8.6	249.6	44.4	100.4	56.7	15.1
Greenville	170,890	86,153	5.7	3.5	14.7	22.3	2.51	137.7	12.3	2.6	8.9	156.0	40.4	89.4	51.6	15.4
Spartanburg	83,215	41,804	4.2	4.0	15.1	28.4	4.41	136.4	5.8	2.1	9.5	173.7	43.1	88.7	54.9	15.0
South Dakota																
Rapid City	43,988	22,138	5.2	3.2	11.5	8.5	3.24	208.4	1.4	2.7	6.9	177.1	29.6	92.2	48.9	19.3
Sioux Falls	235,367	117,471	5.3	5.3	16.2	26.3	3.82	167.5	10.9	2.6	6.6	185.5	32.9	98.5	44.3	14.8
Tennessee																
Chattanooga	145,807	73,291	6.3	4.2	16.0	16.2	1.84	198.2	10.5	1.9	9.0	227.7	41.3	93.3	53.9	12.2
Jackson	92,838	46,308	6.6	3.9	20.0	15.5	4.22	126.5	9.5	2.9	8.9	213.9	46.3	89.5	53.7	13.4
Johnson City	60,397	30,336	4.7	3.8	16.0	13.2	1.94	167.0	15.8	1.6	8.1	214.6	43.7	84.4	52.0	11.4
Kingsport	129,915	65,304	3.9	2.9	14.7	19.3	0.95	170.9	6.8	1.1	8.5	284.3	51.0	80.1	54.8	9.7
Knoxville	295,620	148,780	5.5	4.1	16.9	19.0	2.76	149.7	8.4	2.0	9.4	245.7	45.3	92.3	54.7	13.2
Memphis	370,246	184,400	7.7	5.7	23.1	19.6	2.15	139.5	8.6	2.5	8.7	212.2	46.7	96.7	54.5	13.9
Nashville	473,628	238,276	5.6	3.4	17.7	16.9	3.05	145.5	10.7	3.6	8.9	252.1	40.5	96.6	54.2	13.2
Texas																
Abilene	88,663	44,193	6.4	5.2	16.9	25.4	3.25	157.0	6.8	2.1	8.5	209.4	41.5	94.4	52.2	11.2
Amarillo	103,486	51,880	5.3	3.8	14.0	22.9	2.03	155.6	9.7	4.0	9.1	176.5	30.1	94.7	51.5	13.7
Austin	152,576	76,747	4.9	4.2	16.0	27.5	3.66	157.4	6.9	2.4	8.1	150.7	34.8	87.6	48.6	13.1
Beaumont	116,776	58,697	7.1	5.7	25.7	18.9	2.54	197.8	7.2	2.5	8.4	266.0	46.5	103.5	53.1	17.1
Bryan	36,591	18,365	5.3	4.3	16.1	16.4	2.64	213.1	14.3	4.0	7.8	156.2	32.2	79.0	51.0	5.8
Corpus Christi	106,690	48,764	6.1	4.5	18.0	32.2	1.26	191.3	4.9	2.1	8.0	229.3	41.7	102.4	53.3	19.4
Dallas	570,414	284,100	5.0	6.3	15.3	29.6	2.73	144.9	12.8	2.5	8.9	171.6	35.7	94.8	53.1	13.7
El Paso	149,077	75,702	4.5	3.9	12.9	19.8	1.62	117.5	6.1	2.1	7.1	162.3	38.7	82.2	48.3	14.8
Fort Worth	268,000	133,237	5.2	3.6	12.7	29.7	3.47	142.5	10.5	3.3	9.2	166.5	32.7	91.9	54.7	13.8
Harlingen	75,129	37,984	5.5	5.3	16.6	24.6	0.92	113.9	6.4	1.6	6.6	177.2	42.5	89.6	46.0	10.7
Houston	701,110	354,234	5.4	5.6	18.0	24.3	1.88	165.1	13.4	2.8	8.0	192.5	36.7	99.7	53.0	14.9
Longview	45,796	22,929	4.7	4.0	16.2	32.5	5.31	202.7	12.9	3.6	8.9	190.4	42.5	97.2	51.9	13.5
Lubbock	150,437	75,365	6.2	9.6	31.8	36.7	5.61	184.8	16.7	1.5	9.4	222.3	43.7	120.1	50.9	16.5
McAllen	60,689	30,892	6.7	7.0	21.0	8.3	1.23	143.5	17.6	2.0	6.1	149.2	44.0	94.7	43.7	17.3
Odessa	61,124	30,942	5.3	6.4	16.0	21.0	1.72	91.6	7.1	2.1	9.4	177.7	40.5	95.4	52.6	16.2
San Angelo	41,775	20,900	6.3	4.0	15.5	26.6	2.04	168.7	8.1	5.6	8.1	202.4	38.5	102.2	50.7	15.6
San Antonio	396,618	173,173	4.8	3.1	13.5	19.2	2.21	155.4	10.7	2.1	7.8	178.4	37.4	91.8	50.2	13.9

Hospital Referral Region	Medicare Enrollees (1992 plus 1993)	Medicare Enrollees (1993 only)	CABG Surgery	PTCA	Coronary Angiography (1993)	Prostate Biopsy (1993)	Radical Prostatectomy	Mammography (1993)	Percentage Breast Sparing Surgery	Back Surgery	Hip Fracture	High Variation Medical Conditions	Percentage of Deaths Occurring in Hospitals	All Surgical Discharges	Medicare Mortality	TURP for BPH
Temple	62,494	31,297	4.7	4.0	10.5	14.3	3.26	176.1	13.4	1.6	8.7	162.7	31.6	80.7	50.0	10.0
Tyler	135,417	67,818	5.0	4.8	15.8	27.8	2.91	141.6	5.6	2.6	8.9	196.2	36.7	96.2	50.8	12.6
Victoria	38,195	19,162	4.2	2.6	11.9	10.1	1.69	129.6	9.3	2.3	7.8	238.0	41.3	92.5	48.5	16.2
Waco	85,055	42,325	4.6	3.1	7.9	37.5	2.09	180.1	6.1	2.9	8.5	141.1	32.7	81.3	53.3	14.5
Wichita Falls	57,267	28,594	4.0	3.1	12.6	39.5	4.11	229.9	12.2	2.9	9.4	198.6	40.8	91.8	54.0	18.2
Utah																
Ogden	54,557	27,512	5.4	4.4	12.9	32.0	3.37	133.8	1.9	4.4	6.8	111.0	22.8	84.1	48.0	10.0
Provo	50,865	25,671	6.0	7.3	16.4	34.1	6.66	120.0	5.2	7.0	6.7	118.8	28.8	100.9	45.1	10.4
Salt Lake City	262,005	132,143	4.7	4.2	13.0	24.1	5.58	134.1	16.1	4.0	6.8	115.6	23.3	88.1	46.4	10.3
Vermont																
Burlington	136,818	68,714	5.1	2.9	11.2	22.7	2.04	219.3	26.1	1.9	7.2	197.7	41.1	87.9	52.9	14.6
Virginia																
Arlington	202,392	102,581	3.9	4.1	11.6	20.7	2.31	216.4	22.1	2.9	7.5	165.5	33.2	85.7	49.1	9.2
Charlottesville	112,762	56,899	3.6	3.7	14.0	24.1	2.67	170.3	11.5	2.6	7.5	210.9	36.8	85.8	51.1	9.4
Lynchburg	61,558	30,881	5.3	2.2	13.7	22.6	3.21	161.6	12.8	2.9	8.8	168.9	31.3	85.9	53.7	10.3
Newport News	96,002	48,331	5.5	5.2	20.0	29.2	2.42	251.4	20.2	5.2	7.7	179.9	40.4	100.1	53.0	10.2
Norfolk	218,850	110,305	6.7	4.3	18.1	21.0	1.51	256.5	14.5	3.8	8.1	193.2	42.1	102.4	54.5	11.8
Richmond	301,182	151,733	5.9	6.9	23.6	26.1	3.23	219.2	20.1	3.5	8.0	201.6	39.1	105.5	53.0	10.4
Roanoke	187,728	94,465	5.0	2.8	15.4	17.2	2.36	143.5	16.4	3.0	8.3	227.6	43.5	97.3	53.8	12.4
Winchester	76,789	38,774	5.2	4.3	16.4	13.6	1.86	184.7	8.3	2.7	7.6	238.7	39.0	91.1	55.4	11.3
Washington																
Everett	105,140	44,602	5.3	3.0	9.7	18.5	3.80	195.5	6.5	3.6	7.8	148.4	27.2	87.6	50.8	11.6
Olympia	75,646	34,427	5.0	7.1	17.3	33.8	3.76	229.8	9.0	3.2	7.1	149.4	28.3	91.0	49.1	12.6
Seattle	490,706	207,503	4.7	4.3	10.8	22.3	4.15	249.1	13.5	3.5	7.3	141.0	27.8	87.6	50.3	10.3
Spokane	293,917	146,534	5.2	4.1	12.3	22.3	4.63	211.7	10.9	3.9	7.6	145.3	27.9	89.6	49.4	12.4
Tacoma	123,074	58,974	4.8	2.7	9.6	27.7	3.35	215.6	15.1	4.3	8.0	132.2	27.6	84.3	52.6	11.1
Yakima	57,637	28,649	4.1	3.2	8.8	19.9	4.70	185.3	3.8	3.2	7.5	141.7	30.0	84.9	48.1	16.5
West Virginia																
Charleston	252,516	126,593	6.1	3.9	15.8	16.6	1.52	171.2	10.4	1.5	7.9	254.0	44.6	96.3	55.8	16.9
Huntington	99,385	49,868	4.8	3.9	15.4	25.1	2.12	143.6	10.6	2.0	7.3	253.4	42.3	89.2	58.8	12.5
Morgantown	114,318	57,167	4.9	5.2	19.2	16.0	1.42	196.3	12.7	1.7	7.6	257.0	42.2	96.1	56.3	15.6
Wisconsin																
Appleton	75,703	38,026	4.5	5.2	13.8	26.4	3.88	193.3	11.2	2.3	6.3	147.2	27.0	91.3	49.0	14.0
Green Bay	129,503	64,992	4.4	2.7	9.5	28.8	4.02	228.4	8.1	2.8	6.2	156.7	30.0	91.6	47.8	13.3
La Crosse	96,728	48,299	5.0	3.1	15.5	10.2	4.40	137.1	9.7	1.2	6.9	175.3	28.2	80.9	46.9	9.0
Madison	221,916	111,446	4.8	4.2	13.5	17.6	3.13	168.3	12.7	2.0	7.1	168.9	29.0	91.7	48.2	12.7
Marshfield	106,541	53,474	4.9	3.7	16.3	16.5	3.06	190.8	8.3	1.9	6.6	176.5	30.5	90.3	46.3	10.7
Milwaukee	568,901	284,357	6.2	8.1	22.1	28.3	2.58	174.4	17.1	2.4	6.6	175.4	35.1	98.1	50.9	13.1
Neenah	59,064	29,575	5.7	5.2	17.1	25.1	3.56	217.5	13.3	2.9	6.3	162.7	29.0	95.9	48.2	14.1
Wausau	52,615	26,424	4.8	5.3	15.2	27.2	3.03	183.0	15.3	2.0	6.8	150.4	25.4	92.1	48.5	13.5
Wyoming																
Casper	41,896	21,133	5.1	4.2	10.4	10.8	3.16	172.5	4.9	4.6	7.9	200.8	32.3	94.2	48.9	10.6
United States																
US	61,920,609	294,867,792	5.2	4.9	16.1	25.1	2.76	204.0	16.7	2.7	7.6	190.4	38.7	95.0	51.1	12.9

*All rates are age, sex, and race adjusted. With the exception of "Percentage of Deaths Occurring in Hospitals" and "Percentage Breast Sparing Surgery," rates are per 1,000 enrollees; the rates for surgery are for 1992-93, using a two-year "person-year" denominator as given in the column labeled "Medicare Enrollees (1992 plus 1993)." The apparent discrepancy (e.g., in certain California hospital referral regions) between the two-year and the 1993 counts is explained by the rapid growth of enrollment in risk bearing health maintenance organizations in some hospital referral regions. Rates for mammography and prostate biopsies are for 1993 and are sex-specific. For mammography, prostate biopsy, and coronary angiography, only one procedure per person is counted; i.e., the numerator is individuals with one or more procedures in 1993. To convert to percentages, move the decimal one place to the left. Data exclude Medicare enrollees who are members of risk bearing health maintenance organizations. For benchmarking, two-year Medicare enrollee counts should be used for 1992-93 rates; 1993 counts should be used for 1993 rates. CABG = coronary artery bypass grafting; PTCA = percutaneous transluminal coronary angioplasty. "Percentage Breast Sparing Surgery" is the percentage of all inpatient breast cancer surgery (radical, complete, and partial mastectomies, and lumpectomies) that were partial mastectomies or lumpectomies; "Percentage of Deaths Occurring in Hospitals" is the percentage of all Medicare deaths in hospital referral regions in 1992-93 that occurred in hospitals. TURP for BPH = transurethral prostatectomy for patients with benign prostatic hyperplasia. Specific codes used to define the numerator for rates, and methods of age, sex, and race adjustment are given in Part Nine, Sections 3 and 6.

Description of Variables for Table 4

Variable	Description	Price Adjustment	Figure List
Medicare Population, 1993	The Medicare Population in 1993		
Part A Short Stay Reimbursements	Part A Short Stay Reimbursements per Medicare Enrollee obtained from the 5% CHMS		7.4
Dartmouth Price Adjusted Part A Short Stay Reimbursements	Price Adjusted Part A Short Stay Reimbursements per Medicare Enrollee obtained from the 5% CHMS	Price Index for Medicare Population, 1993	3.2, 4.3, 4.6, 4.7
Part B Reimbursements for Professional and Lab Services	Part B Reimbursement Rates for Professional and Lab Services obtained from the 5% CHMS	Price Index for Medicare Population, 1993	7.4
HCFA Price Adjusted Part B Professional and Lab Services	Price Adjusted Part B Reimbursement Rates for Professional and Lab Services obtained from the 5% CHMS	Price Index for Medicare Population, 1993	4.2, 4.7
HCFA Price Adjusted Part B Medical and Surgical Services	Price Adjusted Part B Reimbursement Rates for Physicians' Medical and Surgical Services obtained from the 5% CHMS		5.4, 5.5
Total Part A and Part B Reimbursements	Total Part A and Part B Reimbursement Rates for all Services obtained from the 5% CHMS		7.4, 7.6
Dartmouth Price Adjusted Total A and B Reimbursements	Price Adjusted Total Part A and Part B Reimbursement Rates for all Services obtained from the 5% CHMS	Price Index for Medicare Population, 1993 was used for the Physician components of the total while the Dartmouth Price Index for Medicare Population, 1993 was used for the rest.	4.1
Home Health Care Reimbursements	Reimbursement Rates for Home Health Care obtained from the 5% CHMS		7.4
Dartmouth Price Adjusted Home Health Care Reimbursements	Price Adjusted Part A Reimbursement Rates for Home Health Care obtained from the 5% CHMS	Price Index for Medicare Population, 1993	4.5
Outpatient Facilities Reimbursements	Reimbursement Rates for Outpatient Facilities obtained from the 5% CHMS		7.4
Dartmouth Price Adjusted Outpatient Facilities Reimbursements	Price Adjusted Part B Reimbursement Rates for Outpatient Facilities obtained from the 5% CHMS	Price Index for Medicare Population, 1993	4.4, 4.6

TABLE FOUR

Unadjusted and Price Adjusted Medicare Reimbursements per Enrollee

by Program Components and Hospital Referral Region (1993)*

Hospital Referral Region	Medicare Enrollees (1993)	Reimbursements for Inpatient Hospital Services	Price Adjusted Reimbursements for Inpatient Hospital Services	Reimbursements for Professional and Lab Services	Price Adjusted Reimbursements for Professional and Lab Services	Price Adjusted Reimbursements for Medical and Surgical Services	Reimbursements for All Services	Price Adjusted Reimbursements for All Services	Reimbursements for Home Health Care Services	Price Adjusted Reimbursements for Home Health Care Services	Reimbursements for Outpatient Facilities	Price Adjusted Reimbursements for Outpatient Facilities
Alabama												
Birmingham	267,273	2,048	2,290	1,059	1,141	644	4,191	4,643	492	550	345	386
Dothan	44,259	1,734	2,041	1,075	1,178	683	3,640	4,199	429	505	272	320
Huntsville	51,975	1,701	1,858	903	962	511	3,438	3,731	326	356	286	312
Mobile	81,643	2,075	2,370	1,070	1,163	662	4,418	4,986	807	921	286	327
Montgomery	48,516	1,716	1,948	1,088	1,172	646	3,744	4,186	461	524	220	250
Tuscaloosa	27,716	1,693	1,951	999	1,080	550	3,449	3,905	397	457	267	307
Alaska												
Anchorage	24,821	2,400	1,995	885	787	469	4,062	3,433	165	137	449	374
Arizona												
Mesa	57,254	1,832	1,844	1,225	1,223	687	3,898	3,911	198	199	289	291
Phoenix	191,774	1,841	1,907	1,161	1,174	657	3,869	3,976	247	256	323	334
Sun City	48,484	1,897	1,910	1,320	1,317	721	3,721	3,733	108	109	189	190
Tucson	86,986	1,637	1,780	1,020	1,044	613	3,641	3,893	267	290	323	351
Arkansas												
Fort Smith	44,277	1,671	2,013	988	1,122	617	3,906	4,636	701	844	233	280
Jonesboro	31,099	1,527	1,958	863	998	539	3,159	3,943	230	295	223	286
Little Rock	193,215	1,683	2,034	927	1,048	558	3,341	3,967	249	301	254	308
Springdale	46,032	1,233	1,538	766	873	478	2,650	3,223	191	239	228	285
Texarkana	35,094	1,654	2,022	907	1,018	547	3,661	4,383	392	479	387	473
California												
Orange Co.	148,733	2,110	1,805	1,580	1,449	866	4,936	4,319	306	262	393	336
Bakersfield	65,463	2,139	2,124	1,406	1,439	884	4,536	4,546	303	301	345	343
Chico	40,695	1,864	1,993	1,030	1,078	673	4,068	4,328	367	392	340	363
Contra Costa Co.	76,593	1,959	1,676	947	874	516	3,810	3,325	252	216	327	280
Fresno	87,954	1,549	1,573	1,068	1,102	657	3,534	3,605	274	278	377	383
Los Angeles	523,261	2,541	2,088	1,738	1,575	946	5,433	4,615	337	277	430	353
Modesto	71,424	2,192	2,213	1,252	1,287	779	4,205	4,268	218	220	288	291
Napa	38,599	2,033	2,036	964	973	651	4,051	4,064	349	349	435	435
Alameda Co.	128,493	2,282	1,921	967	886	545	4,194	3,599	249	209	336	283
Palm Spr/Rancho Mir	33,911	2,108	1,998	1,507	1,482	942	4,729	4,533	179	169	433	410
Redding	41,997	2,137	2,254	1,108	1,159	700	4,249	4,473	373	393	405	427
Sacramento	203,735	2,232	2,121	1,083	1,075	647	4,216	4,052	326	310	298	283
Salinas	32,877	1,866	1,755	1,018	990	641	4,219	4,001	609	572	398	375
San Bernardino	104,442	2,237	2,121	1,367	1,345	811	4,688	4,494	368	349	366	347
San Diego	185,903	2,180	2,039	1,389	1,361	807	4,751	4,505	410	384	352	329
San Francisco	137,196	2,015	1,627	898	798	507	3,974	3,281	300	242	393	318
San Jose	112,354	2,099	1,666	990	877	550	3,931	3,211	229	182	362	288
San Luis Obispo	29,144	1,686	1,586	1,163	1,138	669	3,373	3,215	188	177	214	202

Hospital Referral Region	Medicare Enrollees (1993)	Reimbursements for Inpatient Hospital Services	Price Adjusted Reimbursements for Inpatient Hospital Services	Reimbursements for Professional and Lab Services	Price Adjusted Reimbursements for Professional and Lab Services	Price Adjusted Reimbursements for Medical and Surgical Services	Reimbursements for All Services	Price Adjusted Reimbursements for All Services	Reimbursements for Home Health Care Services	Price Adjusted Reimbursements for Home Health Care Services	Reimbursements for Outpatient Facilities	Price Adjusted Reimbursements for Outpatient Facilities
San Mateo Co.	71,053	1,955	1,541	814	714	480	3,526	2,852	181	143	343	270
Santa Barbara	39,885	1,580	1,434	1,190	1,129	684	3,704	3,412	226	206	295	268
Santa Cruz	24,868	2,183	1,972	1,088	1,021	642	4,283	3,906	483	437	290	262
Santa Rosa	52,191	1,843	1,667	1,053	999	629	3,871	3,548	326	294	278	252
Stockton	42,941	2,118	2,072	1,168	1,170	747	4,141	4,077	174	170	379	371
Ventura	48,138	2,115	1,845	1,499	1,389	826	4,588	4,082	303	265	368	321
Colorado												
Boulder	14,906	1,553	1,609	778	794	442	3,343	3,450	325	336	281	291
Colorado Springs	56,562	1,618	1,798	803	859	468	3,399	3,745	252	280	321	357
Denver	163,270	1,870	1,939	866	893	504	3,779	3,914	329	341	366	380
Fort Collins	23,445	1,795	1,998	894	953	540	3,785	4,171	315	350	428	477
Grand Junction	29,020	1,232	1,472	521	572	300	2,495	2,933	226	271	307	367
Greeley	28,585	1,537	1,750	776	833	482	3,076	3,451	232	264	288	327
Pueblo	19,628	1,612	1,856	757	823	420	3,454	3,928	390	449	302	347
Connecticut												
Bridgeport	88,105	1,743	1,419	1,089	967	560	3,822	3,192	475	386	364	296
Hartford	188,277	1,915	1,647	1,025	946	574	3,913	3,429	342	294	390	335
New Haven	175,454	2,025	1,669	1,138	1,017	599	4,109	3,465	348	287	385	318
Delaware												
Wilmington	73,666	2,321	2,134	1,180	1,144	681	4,228	3,948	224	206	359	330
District of Columbia												
Washington	212,972	2,291	2,068	1,152	1,091	660	4,155	3,803	181	163	388	351
Florida												
Bradenton	48,677	1,676	1,810	1,234	1,243	701	3,610	3,808	269	291	211	228
Clearwater	96,789	1,612	1,715	1,335	1,346	769	3,948	4,127	405	431	201	214
Fort Lauderdale	333,215	1,824	1,755	1,670	1,559	913	4,597	4,375	434	418	351	337
Fort Myers	157,591	1,722	1,903	1,407	1,427	823	4,129	4,427	390	431	305	337
Gainesville	53,306	1,633	1,856	1,131	1,173	637	3,992	4,425	590	671	360	410
Hudson	86,583	1,877	1,998	1,497	1,509	853	4,427	4,621	559	595	254	270
Jacksonville	128,785	1,930	2,102	1,350	1,384	799	4,284	4,579	394	430	347	378
Lakeland	41,935	1,344	1,518	1,073	1,116	640	3,113	3,418	281	317	232	262
Miami	236,134	2,440	2,297	2,635	2,380	1,034	6,429	5,966	650	612	427	401
Ocala	81,014	1,320	1,546	1,218	1,282	697	3,342	3,758	338	396	256	300
Orlando	346,135	1,809	1,932	1,384	1,395	784	4,295	4,501	509	543	285	304
Ormond Beach	45,451	1,696	1,893	1,158	1,190	710	3,827	4,166	400	446	349	389
Panama City	21,241	2,295	2,674	1,427	1,513	862	4,931	5,596	523	609	315	367
Pensacola	71,683	1,914	2,200	1,097	1,163	692	4,161	4,686	564	648	357	410
Sarasota	93,972	1,393	1,509	1,223	1,234	718	3,491	3,689	414	448	241	260
St Petersburg	72,798	1,754	1,867	1,314	1,325	762	4,242	4,443	472	502	311	331
Tallahassee	71,944	1,567	1,787	977	1,035	591	3,526	3,943	340	388	312	355
Tampa	94,672	1,864	1,984	1,301	1,311	744	4,148	4,340	396	422	255	271
Georgia												
Albany	22,092	1,763	2,001	830	892	534	3,394	3,800	416	472	288	327
Atlanta	343,564	2,106	2,147	1,096	1,113	621	4,173	4,250	479	488	321	328
Augusta	61,150	2,066	2,245	1,010	1,070	585	4,126	4,453	412	447	339	369
Columbus	33,178	1,603	1,852	973	1,051	601	3,322	3,767	355	410	248	287

Hospital Referral Region	Medicare Enrollees (1993)	Reimbursements for Inpatient Hospital Services	Price Adjusted Reimbursements for Inpatient Hospital Services	Reimbursements for Professional and Lab Services	Price Adjusted Reimbursements for Professional and Lab Services	Price Adjusted Reimbursements for Medical and Surgical Services	Reimbursements for All Services	Price Adjusted Reimbursements for All Services	Reimbursements for Home Health Care Services	Price Adjusted Reimbursements for Home Health Care Services	Reimbursements for Outpatient Facilities	Price Adjusted Reimbursements for Outpatient Facilities
Macon	72,254	1,863	2,101	983	1,053	555	3,882	4,321	502	566	313	353
Rome	30,054	1,715	2,048	941	1,033	539	3,540	4,137	500	597	284	339
Savannah	68,864	1,813	2,045	961	1,033	578	3,663	4,082	471	532	304	344
Hawaii												
Honolulu	91,283	1,698	1,558	861	794	497	3,175	2,917	151	139	278	255
Idaho												
Boise	68,514	1,258	1,439	666	724	437	2,747	3,105	193	221	308	352
Idaho Falls	16,155	1,644	1,955	711	790	415	3,061	3,588	304	361	294	349
Illinois												
Aurora	16,567	1,836	1,693	762	719	445	3,214	2,980	212	195	292	269
Blue Island	96,480	2,618	2,414	1,177	1,111	698	4,740	4,398	306	282	371	342
Chicago	252,551	2,624	2,420	1,147	1,082	668	4,612	4,272	269	248	329	304
Elgin	40,361	2,420	2,232	1,065	1,004	647	4,481	4,156	288	266	371	342
Evanston	108,566	2,292	2,114	1,189	1,122	692	4,351	4,037	208	192	403	371
Hinsdale	30,199	1,907	1,758	1,156	1,091	634	3,943	3,659	298	274	337	310
Joliet	47,952	2,160	2,118	1,050	1,028	638	3,889	3,811	222	217	309	303
Melrose Park	134,345	2,184	2,014	1,061	1,001	625	4,047	3,755	240	221	276	254
Peoria	94,601	1,561	1,801	838	914	544	3,084	3,506	194	223	329	380
Rockford	85,221	1,621	1,817	873	933	572	3,059	3,384	180	202	266	298
Springfield	129,574	1,671	1,965	807	882	507	3,119	3,600	201	237	276	324
Urbana	56,222	1,455	1,771	775	857	491	2,824	3,350	184	224	280	341
Bloomington	18,958	1,797	2,043	815	881	509	3,280	3,682	133	151	388	441
Indiana												
Evansville	98,732	1,742	2,008	746	828	485	3,443	3,935	350	403	354	408
Fort Wayne	97,436	1,544	1,732	767	838	498	3,044	3,392	256	287	298	334
Gary	56,602	2,520	2,668	1,088	1,160	698	4,572	4,850	364	385	362	383
Indianapolis	285,128	1,860	2,001	833	898	538	3,610	3,886	235	253	381	410
Lafayette	22,767	1,576	1,851	631	701	411	2,985	3,466	245	287	296	348
Muncie	22,925	1,502	1,765	754	846	495	2,841	3,301	118	138	235	276
Munster	40,981	2,577	2,670	1,036	1,092	667	4,588	4,779	293	303	412	427
South Bend	83,059	1,649	1,810	712	767	476	3,025	3,307	173	190	293	322
Terre Haute	27,493	1,795	2,072	743	834	500	3,288	3,773	182	210	251	290
Iowa												
Cedar Rapids	35,134	1,450	1,648	677	732	447	2,657	2,983	91	104	315	358
Davenport	69,196	1,771	2,026	764	836	523	3,229	3,655	165	189	335	383
Des Moines	139,263	1,602	1,884	758	832	503	2,948	3,408	136	160	322	379
Dubuque	21,508	1,428	1,630	521	571	292	2,513	2,844	130	148	313	358
Iowa City	42,355	1,541	1,863	683	756	454	2,786	3,300	128	155	304	368
Mason City	27,052	1,653	2,090	633	718	446	2,899	3,581	153	194	333	421
Sioux City	40,261	1,373	1,693	682	764	450	2,622	3,157	125	155	267	329
Waterloo	32,055	1,558	1,802	596	656	412	2,804	3,211	54	62	413	477
Kansas												
Topeka	55,327	1,459	1,713	745	797	472	2,892	3,320	125	146	308	362
Wichita	173,960	1,760	2,137	905	983	567	3,303	3,895	102	124	361	439
Kentucky												
Covington	36,323	2,025	2,081	893	912	579	3,762	3,862	207	213	271	279

Hospital Referral Region	Medicare Enrollees (1993)	Reimbursements for Inpatient Hospital Services	Price Adjusted Reimbursements for Inpatient Hospital Services	Reimbursements for Professional and Lab Services	Price Adjusted Reimbursements for Professional and Lab Services	Reimbursements for Medical and Surgical Services	Reimbursements for All Services	Price Adjusted Reimbursements for All Services	Reimbursements for Home Health Care Services	Price Adjusted Reimbursements for Home Health Care Services	Reimbursements for Outpatient Facilities	Price Adjusted Reimbursements for Outpatient Facilities
Lexington	149,367	1,725	2,029	871	958	503	3,408	3,943	287	337	294	346
Louisville	184,422	1,943	2,156	1,004	1,084	623	3,897	4,294	275	305	288	320
Owensboro	17,827	1,914	2,285	876	971	579	3,483	4,083	286	341	293	350
Paducah	56,798	1,626	1,993	979	1,097	626	3,314	3,958	240	294	283	347
Louisiana												
Alexandria	33,956	1,988	2,383	969	1,065	564	4,023	4,721	568	681	277	332
Baton Rouge	70,303	2,014	2,259	1,187	1,275	643	4,910	5,446	920	1,032	338	379
Houma	22,428	2,271	2,669	1,350	1,477	791	4,850	5,592	736	865	354	417
Lafayette	57,451	1,972	2,318	1,125	1,235	600	3,926	4,528	386	453	291	342
Lake Charles	25,554	2,251	2,539	935	1,000	552	4,124	4,597	442	499	318	358
Metairie	45,778	2,572	2,701	1,317	1,364	787	5,320	5,569	708	743	419	440
Monroe	33,888	2,072	2,489	1,072	1,180	649	4,574	5,377	803	964	294	353
New Orleans	91,028	2,556	2,623	1,279	1,310	742	5,262	5,391	682	700	395	406
Shreveport	83,987	1,824	2,111	933	1,012	584	3,655	4,161	308	356	345	399
Slidell	15,398	2,682	2,956	1,246	1,332	802	5,139	5,625	427	471	501	552
Maine												
Bangor	54,720	1,618	1,827	733	780	450	2,997	3,336	331	374	270	305
Portland	127,579	1,680	1,788	825	849	507	3,211	3,389	293	312	300	319
Maryland												
Baltimore	274,625	2,803	2,656	1,234	1,200	691	4,890	4,664	203	193	499	473
Salisbury	51,104	2,096	2,240	1,024	1,070	659	3,785	4,020	126	134	360	385
Takoma Park	64,654	2,613	2,239	1,353	1,241	723	4,689	4,100	174	150	376	322
Massachusetts												
Boston	578,227	2,467	2,188	1,086	1,009	569	4,763	4,269	474	420	418	371
Springfield	102,782	2,000	1,972	857	843	510	3,755	3,702	307	303	347	343
Worcester	78,247	2,336	2,061	1,011	938	557	4,417	3,943	409	361	411	362
Michigan												
Ann Arbor	128,729	2,453	2,299	1,277	1,169	677	4,619	4,300	251	235	461	432
Dearborn	72,348	2,283	2,052	1,473	1,296	747	4,677	4,167	274	246	465	418
Detroit	233,448	2,427	2,181	1,480	1,302	730	4,715	4,212	231	208	410	369
Flint	56,620	2,561	2,426	1,408	1,337	715	4,857	4,603	277	263	451	428
Grand Rapids	110,852	1,480	1,545	831	822	472	2,980	3,066	181	189	317	331
Kalamazoo	76,422	1,982	2,073	920	913	521	3,631	3,747	172	180	348	364
Lansing	62,071	1,938	2,020	993	981	577	3,624	3,722	208	217	350	364
Marquette	32,731	1,680	1,890	739	758	465	3,224	3,555	418	470	333	374
Muskegon	34,125	1,413	1,462	797	784	489	2,942	3,003	216	224	365	378
Petoskey	24,459	1,452	1,634	845	866	521	3,078	3,378	288	325	333	375
Pontiac	34,300	2,446	2,199	1,496	1,315	709	4,769	4,253	232	208	441	397
Royal Oak	80,077	2,299	2,066	1,552	1,365	743	4,753	4,240	283	254	439	395
Saginaw	93,134	2,009	2,098	984	980	562	3,736	3,853	224	234	379	396
St Joseph	19,488	1,783	1,910	1,000	1,003	606	3,531	3,714	222	238	356	381
Traverse City	30,614	1,782	2,005	889	912	546	3,417	3,756	255	286	368	415
Minnesota												
Duluth	55,265	1,697	1,891	510	546	328	2,875	3,184	196	218	291	325
Minneapolis	278,212	1,640	1,758	555	585	349	2,794	2,984	95	102	298	319
Rochester	55,172	1,618	1,791	624	671	389	2,639	2,900	46	51	239	265

Hospital Referral Region	Medicare Enrollees (1993)	Reimbursements for Inpatient Hospital Services	Price Adjusted Reimbursements for Inpatient Hospital Services	Reimbursements for Professional and Lab Services	Price Adjusted Reimbursements for Professional and Lab Services	Price Adjusted Reimbursements for Medical and Surgical Services	Reimbursements for All Services	Price Adjusted Reimbursements for All Services	Reimbursements for Home Health Care Services	Price Adjusted Reimbursements for Home Health Care Services	Reimbursements for Outpatient Facilities	Price Adjusted Reimbursements for Outpatient Facilities
St Cloud	25,133	1,411	1,602	595	646	385	2,474	2,779	106	120	251	285
St Paul	71,704	1,754	1,723	605	609	351	3,098	3,057	145	143	326	320
Mississippi												
Gulfport	18,555	2,335	2,639	1,070	1,169	681	4,582	5,142	718	812	327	370
Hattiesburg	31,739	1,927	2,409	1,001	1,136	647	3,812	4,646	526	658	242	302
Jackson	119,625	1,547	1,835	880	971	525	3,503	4,076	598	710	258	306
Meridian	26,687	1,444	1,805	854	969	562	3,063	3,727	371	463	197	246
Oxford	17,195	1,767	2,209	771	875	531	3,533	4,314	598	747	207	259
Tupelo	44,485	1,587	1,981	719	815	483	3,123	3,812	408	509	263	328
Missouri												
Cape Girardeau	38,572	1,344	1,726	708	794	478	2,667	3,311	187	240	333	428
Columbia	88,769	1,802	2,260	767	846	506	3,444	4,203	286	359	387	485
Joplin	52,556	1,580	1,993	750	839	483	3,106	3,810	278	350	325	411
Kansas City	241,129	1,797	1,973	974	1,011	582	3,738	4,045	266	291	371	407
Springfield	106,164	1,568	1,932	762	841	494	3,135	3,764	215	265	380	469
St Louis	418,988	1,947	2,107	877	911	533	3,662	3,924	272	294	348	377
Montana												
Billings	60,821	1,594	1,896	753	827	444	3,010	3,511	179	213	324	386
Great Falls	19,886	1,836	2,225	765	847	454	3,337	3,965	227	275	365	443
Missoula	41,374	1,486	1,816	680	754	425	2,766	3,304	187	228	269	329
Nebraska												
Lincoln	79,126	1,111	1,413	632	723	432	2,208	2,729	100	127	295	375
Omaha	151,270	1,427	1,741	736	827	497	2,814	3,365	157	192	375	458
Nevada												
Las Vegas	86,110	1,889	1,822	1,531	1,512	822	4,488	4,356	501	483	241	232
Reno	59,800	1,667	1,680	1,056	1,059	591	3,531	3,549	264	266	275	277
New Hampshire												
Lebanon	53,424	1,595	1,726	655	679	403	3,022	3,240	322	348	369	399
Manchester	82,822	1,657	1,553	784	750	454	3,133	2,952	237	222	292	273
New Jersey												
Camden	357,129	2,364	2,127	1,275	1,206	730	4,382	4,002	192	173	343	308
Hackensack	158,231	2,050	1,666	1,246	1,113	696	3,936	3,299	167	136	322	262
Morristown	102,808	2,256	1,846	1,214	1,099	660	4,145	3,497	171	140	317	260
New Brunswick	96,187	2,380	1,962	1,231	1,114	670	4,214	3,573	168	139	261	215
Newark	179,074	2,631	2,155	1,260	1,145	725	4,514	3,810	176	144	331	271
Paterson	41,470	2,487	2,019	1,237	1,111	702	4,324	3,616	158	128	279	226
Ridgewood	43,825	2,124	1,747	1,232	1,097	674	4,040	3,407	135	111	337	277
New Mexico												
Albuquerque	117,763	1,256	1,407	756	809	453	2,871	3,178	172	193	384	430
New York												
Albany	240,305	1,667	1,653	941	947	555	3,186	3,173	189	187	256	254
Binghamton	55,190	1,586	1,669	790	827	520	2,935	3,083	166	175	291	306
Bronx	109,294	3,157	2,476	1,362	1,158	726	5,346	4,279	249	195	406	319
Buffalo	210,491	1,568	1,601	880	909	515	3,027	3,100	204	209	276	282
Elmira	55,460	1,787	1,940	898	950	562	3,129	3,371	98	106	275	299
East Long Island	508,296	2,581	2,001	1,461	1,227	736	4,739	3,769	244	189	292	226

Hospital Referral Region	Medicare Enrollees (1993)	Reimbursements for Inpatient Hospital Services	Price Adjusted Reimbursements for Inpatient Hospital Services	Reimbursements for Professional and Lab Services	Price Adjusted Reimbursements for Professional and Lab Services	Price Adjusted Reimbursements for Medical and Surgical Services	Reimbursements for All Services	Price Adjusted Reimbursements for All Services	Reimbursements for Home Health Care Services	Price Adjusted Reimbursements for Home Health Care Services	Reimbursements for Outpatient Facilities	Price Adjusted Reimbursements for Outpatient Facilities
New York	475,687	3,038	2,382	1,558	1,325	789	5,331	4,285	265	208	379	297
Rochester	148,825	1,863	1,855	770	780	456	3,244	3,244	228	227	295	294
Syracuse	134,058	1,825	1,891	898	928	523	3,252	3,366	132	137	265	275
White Plains	131,886	2,359	1,900	1,263	1,090	680	4,214	3,466	162	130	280	226
North Carolina												
Asheville	88,828	1,363	1,597	804	893	520	2,918	3,369	278	326	306	358
Charlotte	187,765	1,763	1,931	848	910	526	3,420	3,726	317	347	306	335
Durham	141,273	1,828	2,057	762	833	486	3,197	3,572	229	258	270	303
Greensboro	61,470	1,901	2,089	843	909	522	3,355	3,671	146	160	245	269
Greenville	80,765	1,751	2,089	823	921	540	3,163	3,713	209	249	272	324
Hickory	29,765	1,996	2,291	813	894	519	3,534	4,023	218	250	281	322
Raleigh	128,251	2,066	2,295	910	986	573	3,742	4,132	281	312	329	366
Wilmington	39,504	1,942	2,176	981	1,066	607	3,810	4,236	414	463	284	318
Winston-Salem	119,943	1,677	1,874	776	844	483	3,091	3,431	176	197	262	292
North Dakota												
Bismarck	30,726	1,717	2,134	709	803	476	3,014	3,668	179	223	316	393
Fargo Moorhead -Mn	72,408	1,476	1,782	596	666	386	2,556	3,032	129	156	230	277
Grand Forks	24,851	1,456	1,774	591	661	396	2,780	3,328	126	153	366	446
Minot	19,663	1,621	2,090	718	825	510	3,005	3,774	126	162	357	460
Ohio												
Akron	88,492	2,202	2,258	998	1,016	608	3,977	4,070	228	234	360	369
Canton	85,218	1,774	1,994	949	1,009	613	3,265	3,611	146	164	252	283
Cincinnati	182,646	2,016	2,099	966	992	604	3,760	3,900	163	170	407	423
Cleveland	287,654	2,275	2,274	1,091	1,097	681	4,176	4,182	220	220	388	388
Columbus	296,162	1,887	2,083	880	925	551	3,451	3,764	183	202	307	339
Dayton	140,131	1,987	2,141	938	978	604	3,586	3,832	168	181	299	322
Elyria	29,207	2,358	2,335	1,155	1,156	753	4,216	4,188	153	151	340	336
Kettering	45,859	1,921	2,003	979	1,004	605	3,624	3,762	210	218	293	306
Toledo	124,817	2,280	2,423	1,044	1,068	671	4,131	4,348	207	220	416	442
Youngstown	115,687	2,417	2,705	1,215	1,295	766	4,388	4,846	223	250	367	411
Oklahoma												
Lawton	24,123	1,629	1,940	785	885	506	2,905	3,409	161	191	250	298
Oklahoma City	204,818	1,770	2,037	867	959	530	3,499	3,988	392	451	271	312
Tulsa	146,680	1,711	1,964	904	998	533	3,545	4,029	473	543	315	361
Oregon												
Bend	18,970	1,549	1,792	822	894	538	3,254	3,710	405	469	262	304
Eugene	84,848	1,431	1,632	824	885	509	2,849	3,194	188	214	240	274
Medford	61,774	1,284	1,423	744	791	465	2,724	2,983	265	294	302	335
Portland	168,475	1,602	1,686	700	729	442	3,120	3,276	221	233	340	357
Salem	28,785	1,424	1,584	700	745	452	2,868	3,157	316	352	252	280
Pennsylvania												
Allentown	153,538	2,291	2,286	1,241	1,255	744	4,372	4,379	275	274	316	316
Altoona	47,695	1,880	2,164	825	901	509	3,727	4,243	379	436	361	416
Danville	78,692	1,904	2,126	906	976	607	3,589	3,972	189	211	415	463
Erie	112,798	1,890	2,141	979	1,060	621	3,651	4,087	220	249	354	401
Harrisburg	124,918	2,103	2,237	988	1,034	616	3,887	4,118	165	176	352	375

Hospital Referral Region	Medicare Enrollees (1993)	Reimbursements for Inpatient Hospital Services	Price Adjusted Reimbursements for Inpatient Hospital Services	Reimbursements for Professional and Lab Services	Price Adjusted Reimbursements for Professional and Lab Services	Price Adjusted Reimbursements for Medical and Surgical Services	Reimbursements for All Services	Price Adjusted Reimbursements for All Services	Reimbursements for Home Health Care Services	Price Adjusted Reimbursements for Home Health Care Services	Reimbursements for Outpatient Facilities	Price Adjusted Reimbursements for Outpatient Facilities
Johnstown	44,399	2,339	2,741	898	996	585	4,176	4,841	296	346	448	525
Lancaster	69,132	1,618	1,662	988	1,006	622	3,220	3,298	116	120	353	363
Philadelphia	522,192	2,624	2,379	1,392	1,309	784	4,837	4,434	204	185	368	333
Pittsburgh	523,354	2,669	2,786	1,180	1,239	719	4,873	5,096	356	372	390	407
Reading	85,239	1,782	1,851	1,001	1,035	633	3,511	3,642	187	195	277	287
Sayre	28,008	1,890	2,129	747	805	496	3,201	3,572	178	200	253	285
Scranton	58,229	1,889	2,072	1,138	1,220	724	4,129	4,501	420	461	285	313
Wilkes-Barre	49,540	2,061	2,245	1,199	1,282	764	4,447	4,821	447	487	356	388
York	47,991	1,517	1,629	840	884	553	3,016	3,221	162	174	272	292
Rhode Island												
Providence	152,455	2,084	1,930	1,011	946	541	3,997	3,711	374	346	343	318
South Carolina												
Charleston	76,139	1,898	2,109	954	1,042	624	3,751	4,150	322	358	363	404
Columbia	108,229	1,553	1,742	818	900	518	2,986	3,331	226	253	233	261
Florence	38,625	1,926	2,226	932	1,038	573	3,554	4,068	256	296	290	335
Greenville	86,153	1,791	1,988	826	908	510	3,321	3,678	192	213	314	349
Spartanburg	41,804	1,646	1,837	795	875	492	3,092	3,439	232	259	289	323
South Dakota												
Rapid City	22,138	1,267	1,599	617	706	407	2,456	3,027	206	260	226	286
Sioux Falls	117,471	1,410	1,798	646	738	425	2,492	3,092	71	90	273	348
Tennessee												
Chattanooga	73,291	1,942	2,132	921	998	539	4,639	5,081	1,177	1,292	378	415
Jackson	46,308	1,746	2,069	924	1,034	576	3,891	4,548	722	856	354	419
Johnson City	30,336	1,865	2,142	829	920	497	3,689	4,208	547	629	282	324
Kingsport	65,304	1,979	2,274	801	888	470	3,714	4,240	445	511	293	337
Knoxville	148,780	1,855	2,116	895	988	547	4,006	4,542	855	975	297	339
Memphis	184,400	1,878	2,132	968	1,058	600	3,749	4,209	506	574	243	276
Nashville	238,276	1,940	2,205	900	984	525	4,245	4,785	850	966	314	357
Texas												
Abilene	44,193	1,705	2,051	883	980	526	3,561	4,200	514	619	282	340
Amarillo	51,880	1,639	1,887	864	941	512	3,429	3,895	461	530	266	307
Austin	76,747	1,466	1,536	965	992	541	3,454	3,600	383	401	269	282
Beaumont	58,697	2,447	2,644	1,272	1,321	701	5,145	5,505	714	771	333	360
Bryan	18,365	1,551	1,855	915	1,000	501	3,230	3,772	284	340	300	359
Corpus Christi	48,764	2,369	2,650	1,213	1,305	734	4,986	5,528	711	795	336	375
Dallas	284,100	1,812	1,863	1,086	1,112	589	3,997	4,105	399	411	356	366
El Paso	75,702	1,703	1,937	936	1,010	544	3,597	4,037	353	401	317	360
Fort Worth	133,237	1,840	1,953	1,007	1,043	540	4,038	4,261	415	441	303	321
Harlingen	37,984	2,410	2,889	1,069	1,181	653	4,373	5,145	435	521	333	399
Houston	354,234	2,331	2,347	1,173	1,170	660	4,603	4,624	348	350	421	423
Longview	22,929	1,961	2,243	1,000	1,089	583	3,773	4,262	348	398	349	399
Lubbock	75,365	2,097	2,496	1,129	1,236	677	4,160	4,844	387	460	370	441
McAllen	30,892	1,961	2,332	1,145	1,266	634	3,912	4,553	357	425	339	403
Odessa	30,942	1,966	2,167	1,085	1,163	640	4,009	4,389	427	471	258	285
San Angelo	20,900	1,800	2,207	954	1,061	588	3,467	4,143	276	339	317	389
San Antonio	173,173	1,700	1,906	1,111	1,190	635	3,992	4,420	525	589	372	417

Hospital Referral Region	Medicare Enrollees (1993)	Reimbursements for Inpatient Hospital Services	Price Adjusted Reimbursements for Inpatient Hospital Services	Reimbursements for Professional and Lab Services	Price Adjusted Reimbursements for Professional and Lab Services	Price Adjusted Reimbursements for Medical and Surgical Services	Reimbursements for All Services	Price Adjusted Reimbursements for All Services	Reimbursements for Home Health Care Services	Price Adjusted Reimbursements for Home Health Care Services	Reimbursements for Outpatient Facilities	Price Adjusted Reimbursements for Outpatient Facilities
Temple	31,297	1,687	1,916	620	667	346	3,014	3,386	228	259	328	372
Tyler	67,818	1,775	2,070	1,045	1,142	593	3,896	4,468	406	474	422	492
Victoria	19,162	1,607	1,813	819	889	488	3,151	3,521	265	299	281	318
Waco	42,325	1,282	1,505	741	811	421	2,673	3,082	194	228	289	339
Wichita Falls	28,594	1,522	1,848	951	1,054	545	3,488	4,135	398	483	276	335
Utah												
Ogden	27,512	1,617	1,764	645	693	394	3,141	3,422	422	461	266	291
Provo	25,671	1,862	2,194	745	824	485	3,545	4,127	412	486	313	369
Salt Lake City	132,143	1,482	1,655	691	748	401	3,080	3,419	418	467	287	320
Vermont												
Burlington	68,714	1,797	1,935	741	776	503	3,204	3,429	219	235	361	389
Virginia												
Arlington	102,581	1,800	1,543	1,086	996	584	3,680	3,218	244	209	352	302
Charlottesville	56,899	1,820	1,973	764	812	484	3,245	3,502	149	162	371	402
Lynchburg	30,881	1,548	1,712	620	673	435	2,562	2,821	95	105	222	245
Newport News	48,331	1,508	1,586	911	959	604	3,109	3,270	217	228	323	340
Norfolk	110,305	1,908	2,050	1,037	1,105	668	3,647	3,909	205	220	344	370
Richmond	151,733	1,802	1,794	930	953	569	3,321	3,335	162	162	318	316
Roanoke	94,465	1,704	1,941	768	841	481	3,189	3,599	245	279	311	354
Winchester	38,774	1,794	1,857	727	749	450	3,135	3,243	158	164	307	318
Washington												
Everett	44,602	1,627	1,664	826	840	496	3,328	3,399	244	249	404	413
Olympia	34,427	1,854	1,972	922	959	552	3,635	3,844	284	302	334	356
Seattle	207,503	1,661	1,650	887	886	501	3,387	3,370	231	230	325	323
Spokane	146,534	1,605	1,769	860	916	512	3,155	3,445	186	205	300	330
Tacoma	58,974	1,642	1,691	895	915	528	3,334	3,427	196	201	317	326
Yakima	28,649	1,455	1,601	853	901	496	2,960	3,218	191	210	312	344
West Virginia												
Charleston	126,593	1,938	2,251	802	869	500	3,427	3,920	217	252	292	340
Huntington	49,868	2,000	2,286	933	1,009	584	3,611	4,072	165	189	218	249
Morgantown	57,167	2,027	2,444	814	896	516	3,698	4,374	223	269	349	421
Wisconsin												
Appleton	38,026	1,352	1,527	621	657	413	2,491	2,770	59	67	283	320
Green Bay	64,992	1,502	1,704	718	759	456	2,807	3,127	117	133	321	365
La Crosse	48,299	1,417	1,664	578	626	373	2,424	2,793	123	144	215	252
Madison	111,446	1,600	1,779	643	671	389	2,871	3,148	172	192	254	282
Marshfield	53,474	1,501	1,764	727	782	451	2,744	3,154	199	233	200	235
Milwaukee	284,357	1,909	1,952	886	892	542	3,477	3,542	134	137	327	335
Neenah	29,575	1,450	1,633	685	724	440	2,718	3,013	104	117	309	348
Wausau	26,424	1,234	1,431	766	819	503	2,618	2,966	159	184	268	311
Wyoming												
Casper	21,133	1,977	2,269	781	848	447	3,584	4,069	366	420	322	370
United States												
US	29,486,792	1,985	2,018	1,055	1,057	613	3,901	3,962	302	313	333	342

*The data are age, sex, and race adjusted for Medicare enrollees who were not members of risk bearing health maintenance organizations on June 30, 1993. See Part Nine, Section 4, for details on constructing rates and adjusting for price.

PART NINE

Strategies and Methods

1. The Geography of Health Care in The United States

1.1 Files Used in the Atlas

The Atlas depends on the integrated use of a large number of databases provided by the American Hospital Association (AHA), the American Medical Association, the American Osteopathic Association, and several federal agencies, including the Agency for Health Care Policy and Research, the Bureau of the Census, the Health Care Financing Administration, the National Center for Health Statistics, and the Department of Veterans Affairs. Table 1 lists these files and provides a short description of the uses made of them in the Atlas.

Table 1. Data Files Used in Analysis

File	Year Used (Sample)	Source / Provider	Description and Use in Analyses
Medicare Files			
Denominator File	1992 & 1993 (100%)	HCFA	Contains one record for each Medicare beneficiary, and includes demographic information (age, sex, race), residence (ZIP Code), program eligibility and mortality. Used to determine denominators for utilization and expenditure rates and to determine mortality.
MEDPAR File	1992 & 1993 (100%)	HCFA	One record for each hospital stay by Medicare beneficiaries. Includes data on dates of admission / discharge, diagnoses, procedures and Medicare reimbursements to the hospital. Used for (1) defining health care markets (2) allocation of acute care resources and physicians, (3) numerators for utilization rates.
Part B File	1993 (5%)	HCFA	Contains records of physician and supplier claims submitted under the Part B program. Physician records include a beneficiary identifier, dates, procedure codes and payments. Used to define numerators for certain procedure rates.
Continuous Medicare History Sample File	1993 (5%)	HCFA	Includes a record for each beneficiary in a 5% sample for each year. Includes summary expenditure data. Used to estimate Medicare spending by program component.
Medicare Provider of Services File	1993	HCFA	Includes a record for each hospital eligible to provide inpatient care through Medicare. Includes location and resource data. Used in measuring acute care resource investments.
Medicare Cost Reports	1991 & 1992	HCFA	Includes a record for each hospital and provides detailed accounting data for the specified year. Used in measuring acute care resource investments.

File	Year Used	Source/Provider	Description and Use in Analyses
Resource Files			
American Hospital Association Annual Survey of Hospitals	1993	American Hospital Association	Includes a record for each hospital registered with the AHA. Used in measuring acute care resources (beds, personnel, expenditures).
Physician File	1993	American Medical Association	Includes one record for each allopathic physician with practice ZIP Code, self-designated specialty, major professional activities, and federal / non-federal status. Used to determine specialty-specific counts of physicians in each health care market.
Osteopath File	1993	American Osteopathic Association	Includes one record for each osteopathic physician with practice ZIP Code, self-designated specialty, major professional activities, and federal / non-federal status. Used to determine specialty-specific counts of physicians in each health care market.
Federal hospital utilization and resources	1993-1994	U.S. Medicine Directory 1993-94 ISSN 0890-6637	Provides location, counts and occupancy rates of federal hospital beds.
VA patient travel pattern file	1989	VA Outcomes Group, White River Jct VA	ZIP Code level patient origin file for veterans using VA hospitals in 1989. Used to allocate VA physicians to appropriate HSAs.
Other Files			
Geographic Practice Cost Index	1993	HCFA	Records for each MSA and non-MSA area of each state. Records include area-level values for each of the components of the GPCI (physician work, practice cost, malpractice) and summary index value. Used for price adjustment.
National Hospital Discharge Survey	1989	NTIS	Provides age-sex specific hospital discharge rates for the U.S. as a whole, which were used as the basis for the age-sex adjustment of acute care resources.
National Ambulatory Medical Care Survey (NAMCS)	1989-1992	NTIS	Ambulatory services from samples of patient records selected from a national sample of office-based physicians. Allows estimation of age-sex specific use rates by specialty. Used for age-sex adjustment of physician workforce.
Population files	1990	Claritas, Inc., Arlington, VA	1990 STF3 data from the U.S. Bureau of the Census was adapted by Claritas, Inc. to 1993 ZIP Code geography; includes age-sex specific counts of residents in the ZIP Code. Used (1) for age-sex adjustment, (2) as denominator for rates of allocated and adjusted resources.
ZIP Code boundary files	1993	Geographic Data Technology, Lebanon, NH	Includes records for each ZIP Code with the coordinates of the boundary precisely specified. Used as basis for mapping HSAs and HRRs and for assigning ZIP Codes appropriately.

1.2 Defining Hospital Service Areas

Hospital Service Areas (HSAs) represent local health care markets for community-based inpatient care. HSAs were defined in three steps. First, all acute care hospitals in the 50 states and the District of Columbia were identified from the American Hospital Association Annual Survey of Hospitals and the Medicare Provider of Services files and assigned to a location within a town or city. The list of towns or cities with at least one acute care hospital (N=3,953) defined the maximum number of possible HSAs. Second, all 1992 and 1993 acute care hospitalizations of the Medicare population were analyzed according to ZIP Code to determine the proportion of residents' hospital stays that occurred in each of the 3,953 candidate HSAs. ZIP Codes were initially assigned to the HSA where the greatest proportion (plurality) of residents were hospitalized. Approximately 500 of the candidate HSAs did not qualify as independent HSAs because the plurality of patients resident in those HSAs were hospitalized in other HSAs.

The third step required visual examination of the ZIP Codes used to define each HSA. Maps of ZIP Code boundaries were made using files obtained from Geographic Data Technologies (GDT) and each HSA's component ZIP Codes were examined. In order to achieve contiguity of the component ZIP Codes for each HSA, "island" ZIP Codes were reassigned to the enclosing HSA, and/or HSAs were grouped into larger HSAs . (See Part One for an illustration.) Certain ZIP Codes used in the Medicare files were restricted in their use to specific institutions (e.g., a nursing home) or a post office. These "point ZIPs" were assigned to their enclosing ZIP Code based on the ZIP Code boundary map.

This process resulted in the identification of 3,436 HSAs, ranging in total population from 866 (Hoven, South Dakota) to 2,680,712 (Chicago, Illinois). In most HSAs, the majority of Medicare hospitalizations occurred in a hospital or hospitals located within the HSA. See Part One for further details.

1.3 Defining Hospital Referral Regions

Hospital referral regions (HRRs) represent health care markets for tertiary medical care. As defined here, each HRR contained at least one HSA that had a hospital or hospitals that performed major cardiovascular procedures and neurosurgery in 1992-93. Three steps were taken to define HRRs.

First, the candidate hospitals and HRRs were identified. A total of 862 hospitals performed at least 10 major cardiovascular procedures (DRGs 103-107) on Medicare enrollees in both years. These hospitals were located within 458 HSAs, thereby defining the maximum number of possible HRRs. Further checks verified that all 458 HSAs included at least one hospital performing the specified major neurosurgical procedures (DRGs 1-3 and 484).

Second, we calculated in each of the 3,436 HSAs in the United States the proportion of major cardiovascular procedures performed in each of the 458 candidate HRRs in 1992-93. Each HSA was then assigned provisionally to the candidate HRR where most patients went for these services.

Third, HSAs were reassigned or further grouped to achieve (a) geographic contiguity, unless major travel routes (e.g., interstate highways) justified separation (this occurred in only two cases, the New Haven, Connecticut, and Elmira, New York, HRRs); (b) a minimum population size of 120,000; and (c) a high localization index – at least 65% of all the hospitalizations of HRR patients were to hospitals located within the HRR. Because of the large number of hospitals providing cardiovascular services in California, several candidate California HRRs met the above criteria but were found to perform small numbers of cardiovascular procedures. These HRRs were further aggregated according to county boundaries to achieve stability of cardiovascular surgery rates within the areas.

The process resulted in the definition of 306 hospital referral regions which ranged in size from 121,666 (Bend, Oregon) to 8,891,233 (Los Angeles). See Part One for further details.

1.4 Populations of HSAs and HRRs

Total population counts were estimated for residents of all ages in each HSA using ZIP Code level files obtained from Claritas, Inc. The Claritas file is based on the 1990 U.S. Census STF3B ZIP Code file, updated to account for changes in ZIP Code definitions. Population counts for HRRs are the sum of the counts of the constituent HSAs. These serve as the denominator for estimating rates for hospital and physician workforce allocations (Part Two and Part Five). For rates that apply to the Medicare population for the years 1992-93 (Parts Three and Six), enrollee counts were obtained from the Medicare Denominator file. The 1992 and 1993 Medicare enrollee population included those alive and age 65 to age 99 on June 30, 1992 and 1993, respectively. For Medicare reimbursement rates (Part Four), and for diagnostic procedure rates based on Part B claims (Part Six), the enrollee counts are based on a 5% sample of Medicare enrollees for 1993 (selected on the basis of Social Security numbers that end in 05, 20, 45, 70 or 95). For most of the rates presented in this analysis, the numerator and the denominator counts exclude those who were enrolled in risk bearing HMOs on June 30.

Acute care resources consist of hospital beds, personnel and expenditures. Three tasks were required to estimate the rates presented in Part Two. First, the resources for each hospital had to be determined; second, resources had to be allocated to populations, proportionate to their rates of use; third, rates had to be constructed and adjusted to take into account differences in age, sex and, in the case of expenditures, the price of care, between regions.

2. Hospital Resource Rates

2.1 Measuring Hospital Resources

Hospitals were eligible for inclusion if they were located within the 50 states or the District of Columbia and were classified either by Medicare or the AHA as short term general medical and surgical hospitals (AHA service code = 10), specialty hospitals listed as obstetrics and gynecology (code 44), eye, ear, nose and throat (code 45), orthopedic (code 47), or other specialty (code 49); and children's hospitals (codes 50,59). For inclusion in this study, hospitals must have been open on June 30, 1993. Certain specialty hospitals were excluded if additional information gathered from external sources (e.g., telephone calls) indicated they did not meet the inclusion criteria, or if they fell into the following categories: Shriners' hospitals, crippled children's hospitals, hospital units of institutions (prisons, colleges, etc.), institutions for mental retardation, psychiatric facilities, rehabilitation or chronic disease facilities, addiction treatment facilities, communication disorders facilities, podiatry facilities, small surgery centers, obstetrics and gynecology clinics, and hospices. Department of Veterans' Affairs hospitals were excluded from this edition of the Atlas because of the non-comparability of expenditure and personnel data.

The American Hospital Association Annual Survey file and the Medicare Provider file were searched to identify all non-federal hospitals (AHA control code = 12-33) and federal PHS Indian Service hospitals (control code = 47) that met the criteria for inclusion. Short term general hospitals (N= 5,075), children's hospitals (N=53), and specialty hospitals (N=65) located in the 50 states or the District of Columbia as of June 30, 1993 were identified.

The resources for each hospital were determined as follows:

Hospital beds were ascertained primarily from the AHA file. The field selected was "hospital beds (including cribs, pediatric and neonatal bassinets) that were set up and staffed at the end of the reporting period." For the 30 hospitals completely lacking AHA data, and for the 378 hospitals that were non-reporting in 1993, we used data from the Medicare Cost Reports for "total beds available in the hospital." The remaining 15 non-reporting hospitals (all PHS Indian Service hospitals) also lacked cost report data, so AHA data were used to measure all resources, even though the data came from a prior year's Annual Survey.

Full time equivalent hospital personnel were defined as the sum of full time employees and 1/2 of the part time employees. Hospital employees do not include medical or dental interns or residents or trainees. For the 30 hospitals lacking AHA data completely and for 378 of the 392 hospitals that were non-reporting in 1993, the Medicare Cost Report value for "average number of employees, hospital total" was used to estimate hospital personnel at these hospitals.

Full time equivalent registered nurses were defined as the sum of full time nurses and 1/2 of the part time nurses. For the 30 hospitals lacking AHA data completely and for 378 of the 392 hospitals that were non-reporting for 1993, the Medicare Provider of Services file count of "licensed registered nurses" was used to estimate the number of registered nurses at these hospitals.

Hospital expenditures were defined using the 1993 AHA Annual Survey estimate of total hospital expenses, which includes both payroll and non-payroll components, plus non-operating losses (where payroll expenses include all salaries and wages except those paid to medical and dental interns and residents and other trainees, e.g., medical technology trainees, X-ray therapy trainees, administrative residents, etc.). For the 30 hospitals lacking AHA data, and for 378 of the 392 non-reporting hospitals, total facility costs were estimated from Medicare Cost Report data (and were annualized where necessary).

2.2 Allocation of Hospital Resources

In order to account for the use of care by patients who live in one HSA but obtain care in another, hospital resources for acute care short-term hospitals have been allocated to the HSAs in proportion to the actual patterns of use. This was accomplished using the proportion of all Medicare patient days (1992-93) provided by each specific hospital to each HSA. For example, if 60% of total Medicare inpatient days at a hospital were used by residents of the HSA where the hospital was located, then 60% of that hospital's resources would be assigned to its HSA. If 20% of the Medicare patient days provided by that hospital were used by a neighboring HSA, 20% of the hospital's resources would be assigned to that neighboring HSA.

Children's hospitals and specialty hospitals were found to have too little actual utilization data in the Medicare files to allow their allocation based on hospital-specific proportionate utilization. These hospitals were allocated according to the utilization patterns of all Medicare enrollees residing in the HSA. In other words, if 80% of the patient days in an HSA were provided by hospitals within the HSA, then 80% of the resources of any specialty or children's hospital located within that HSA would be assigned to it.

The use of Medicare data to estimate resources allocated to populations of all ages is justified by studies which show that the geographic patterns of use of hospital care by patients under and over sixty-five years of age are similar. Our own analyses of data from both New York and New England revealed that travel patterns for those under age 65 are nearly identical to those over age 65. Radany and Luft (1993) found similar results in California.

Once each of the hospital resources had been allocated to HSAs, the allocated resources were summed. For example, the allocated beds of each HSA were equal to the sum of allocated acute short-term beds and allocated specialty/children's beds. For the HSAs located in a given HRR, resources were further summed to obtain the total for the HRR. Crude rates were then calculated for HRRs using the 1990 population for all ages described in section 1.4.

2.3 Calculation of Adjusted Per Capita Resources

The resource allocation rates presented in Part Two of the Atlas were adjusted for differences in age and sex using the indirect method. Since the national age-sex specific bed supply rates are not available, these were estimated using the national age and sex specific patient day rates obtained from the 1989 National Hospital Discharge Survey. These estimates were used to calculate the expected bed supply in each HRR. Under the assumption that expenditures and employee allocations across age and sex groups are also proportionate to patient days, a similar strategy was used to adjust expenditures and employees.

Hospital expenditure rates were further adjusted to account for regional differences in prices. Seeking to avoid a price adjustment that depended on physician or hospital market conditions, we focused on cost of living indices using non-medical regional price measures. We used the Geographic Practice Cost Index (GPCI) applicable to fiscal year 1995 Medicare physician claims. The index is the weighted sum of three components: the relative cost of non-physician professional labor across areas, the relative cost of physician practice inputs (principally rents and wages to office employees) and the relative cost of malpractice. The weights are based on the national proportions of these costs in physician services. We reweighted the index, excluding the malpractice costs. We also used the full professional labor component in our revised index (HCFA used only one-quarter of the professional labor component). While not perfectly exogenous to health care (as it includes physician office expenses), the GPCI is both available at the level of geographic analysis needed in this study, and is preferable to the major alternative, Medicare's hospital wage index. (The hospital wage index is based on actual wages paid to hospital employees in each area and is thus distorted by differences in occupational mix and market conditions. Hospitals that hire more highly paid staff have those costs reflected in the wage index.) The GPCI is discussed in greater detail by the originators of the measure, Zuckerman, Welch and Pope (1990).

The modified GPCI (exclusive of malpractice costs) was available for each metropolitan statistical area (MSA) and for non-MSA areas of each state. The values for the area-specific modified GPCI were assigned to each HSA according to the location of the principal city or town of each HSA.

To calculate HRR-level modified GPCIs, we calculated weighted sums of the HSA-specific index, using the general population size of the HSA as the weight. The index was then applied to adjust the allocated hospital expenditures. Area-specific allocated expenditures were divided by the index for that area. New York's modified GPCI was 1.275, indicating that costs in that area are 27.5% higher than the national average. Allocated hospital expenditures per capita for New York were $1,871. Dividing by New York's modified GPCI gives an adjusted per capita expenditure of $1,467, which is the figure presented in the maps and tables.

Adjusting for differences in the price level shifts the relative rankings of hospital referral regions, in some cases by a large amount. Consider, for example, inpatient acute care hospital expenditures. Table Two displays the per capita acute care hospital expenditures for three hospital referral regions: Anchorage, Alaska, Lincoln, Nebraska, and the Bronx, New York. Both unadjusted data and data after price adjustment are included. In the case of Anchorage, the unadjusted measure of acute care costs led to a ranking of 13th in the country, with average expenditures of $798. After adjustment for the much higher cost of living in Anchorage, its rank drops to 95th, with spending of $662. By contrast, adjusting for the lower average prices in the Lincoln hospital referral region raises its relative ranking from 284th to 233rd. Sometimes price adjustment makes little difference in the relative ranking. Even after average acute care inpatient expenses in the Bronx hospital referral region are adjusted downward from $1,266 to $993, it still ranks first in total expenditures per resident.

Table 2. Acute Care Hospital Expenditures per Person, Adjusted for Price Differences

Location	Unadjusted Expenditures	Unadjusted Rank	Adjusted Expenditures	Adjusted Rank
Anchorage, Alaska	$798	13	$662	95
Lincoln, Nebraska	$432	284	$540	233
The Bronx, New York	$1,266	1	$993	1

2.4 The Distribution Graph

The distribution graphs used in the Atlas provide a simple way to show the dispersion in particular rates of health care resources and utilization across the 306 hospital referral regions. For example, the graph below shows the distribution of hospital beds per thousand residents for each of the 306 hospital referral regions. The vertical axis shows the rate of hospital beds per thousand residents. The highest point in the graph represents the hospital referral region with the largest number of hospital beds per capita, Monroe, Louisiana, which has 5.3 beds per thousand residents. Bismarck, North Dakota, and New Orleans, Louisiana, which both have 5.2 beds per thousand, are represented by the next two points on the graph. Some areas which do not have precisely the same number of hospital beds per thousand residents are arrayed on a single line because their rates fall into a "bin" between two values.

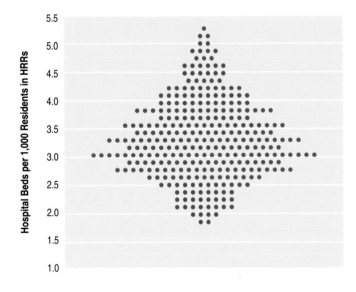

This chart summarizes two features of the data. The first is a measure of dispersion; if the number of beds per thousand (or whatever measure is on the vertical axis) for the highest hospital referral region is two or three times the number of beds per thousand for the lowest hospital referral region, it suggests substantial variation in health care resources. Second, the distribution graph shows whether the variation is caused by just a few outliers – hospital referral regions that for various reasons are much different from the rest of the country – or whether the variation is pervasive and widespread across the country. In the example above, the dispersion is not caused by just a few areas such as Monroe and Bismarck; there is widespread dispersion.

3. Hospital Utilization Rates

Rates represent counts of the number of events that occurred in a defined time period (the numerator) for a specific population (the denominator). The rates in Part Three are for 1992 and 1993. The counts of events are based on the MEDPAR files for 1992-93. The denominator is the 1992-93 Medicare enrollee population (Section 1.4). In order to assure that the events counted in the numerator correspond to the denominator population, certain records were excluded, including Medicare enrollees who were under age 65 or over age 99 on June 30, 1992 or 1993; Medicare enrollees who were enrolled in risk-bearing HMOs; MEDPAR records with a length of stay over 365 days; hospitalizations in psychiatric, rehabilitation or long term care units (provider codes = S, T, U or V; facility type not equal to S; third digit of Medicare provider number not equal to 0).

3.1 Conditions examined in Part Three of the Atlas

The specific conditions or "numerator events" presented in Part Three, the data files used to generate the counts, and the codes used to identify the event in the file are given in Table 3.

Table 3. Definitions for Categories of Events in Part Three of the Atlas

Condition	Source File	Codes used to define condition
All discharges	MEDPAR	All records for eligible enrollees
In-hospital deaths	MEDPAR	Discharge status = B
Hip fracture	MEDPAR	Principal diagnosis = ICD 820.0 - 820.99
Surgical admissions	MEDPAR	See Note 1
High variation medical conditions	MEDPAR	See Note 2
Percent dying in hospital	MEDPAR	In-hospital deaths / all deaths in HRR
Deaths	Denominator	Eligible enrollees with date of death 1/1/92 - 12/31/93

NOTES:

1. Surgical DRGs are the following: 1-8, 36-42, 49-63, 75-77, 103-108, 110-120, 146-171, 191-201, 209-234, 257-270, 285-293, 302-315, 334-345, 353-365, 370, 371, 377, 392-394, 400-402, 406-408, 415, 424, 439-443, 458, 459, 461, 468, 471-472, 476-486, 488, 491, 493, 494

2. HVMC are those with the following DRGs: 9-13, 15-35, 43-48, 64-74, 78-102, 124-145, 172-173, 176-190, 202-208, 235-256, 271-284, 294-301, 316-333, 346-352, 366-369, 372, 373, 376, 378-391, 395-399, 403-405, 409-414, 416-423, 425-437, 444-457, 460, 462-467, 473, 475, 487, 489, 490, 492

3.2 Calculation of Adjusted Procedure and Mortality Rates

The denominator for inpatient utilization and mortality rates was the Medicare enrollee population resident in HRRs in 1992-93 (Section 1.4). The denominator for determining the percentage dying in hospital was the count of all deaths among Medicare enrollees resident in HRRs in 1992-93, obtained from the Medicare Denominator File. Rates were adjusted using the indirect method for the following strata: sex, race (black, non-black) and age (65-69, 70-74, 75-79, 80-84, 85-89, 90-94, 95-99).

Although standard errors of the rates were not reported, these estimates are, for the most part, precisely determined. The minimum Medicare population in an HRR is 14,000 residents, and all rates were based on a count of at least 15 events. The following precisions were obtained in this "worst case scenario" for an event rate of 5 per 1,000:

- For procedures related exclusively to males or females in this smallest HRR, the precision would be ±17% of the true rate.
- For procedures related to the entire HRR, the precision would be ±12%.
- For procedures in a median-sized HRR (N=65,000) the precision would be ±6%.

In general, if we denote the event rate as p and the population size as N, the standard error is $\sqrt{(p/N)}$ and the precision expressed as a percent of the true rate is $(p/se(p))*100\%$.

Although the majority of events occurred at most once per person during the study period, we included multiple events to the same person to allow the rates to reflect total health care utilization.

3.3 Measures of Association (R^2 and Regression Lines)

In this Atlas, we often suggest that some factors may be related in a systematic way to other factors. For example, in Part Three we hypothesize that regions with high ratios of beds per thousand residents also have high rates of hospital expenditures.

To capture the degree and extent of the correlation between hospital beds and expenditures in Figure 3.1, we put hospital beds per thousand residents on the horizontal axis and hospital expenditures per capita on the vertical axis, and placed a point on the graph for each of the 306 hospital referral regions. If hospital beds and expenditures were negatively correlated, so that regions with higher beds per thousand residents had lower per capita expenditures, then we might expect to see the cloud of points tilted downward, running from northwest to southeast. Conversely, if they were positively correlated – as they in fact are – the cloud of points would run from southwest to northeast on the graph, as seen in Figure 3.1.

It is sometimes difficult to discern from this cloud of points the relationship between two variables. A linear regression line provides the best fit of the data and summarizes the relationships between them. A measure of the "goodness of fit" or the extent to which hospital beds per 1,000 predicts expenditures per capita is the R^2, which is defined as the fraction of total variation in the vertical axis (expenditures) that is explained by variation in the horizontal axis (beds). It can range between 0 and 1, where 1 is perfect correlation and 0 means that the two variables are completely unrelated. In Figure 3.1, the R^2 is .57, which means that the two are closely related – that 57% of the variation in price, age, and sex adjusted expenditures per capita is related to the age and sex adjusted bed supply.

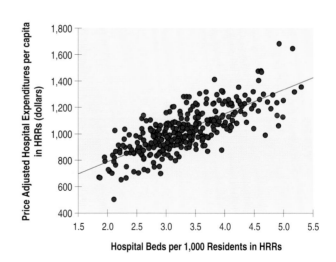

The regression lines and R^2 statistics given in the text are not weighted for the size of the population. Weighted and unweighted R^2 statistics were similar.

4. Medicare Program Reimbursement Rates

The numerators for Medicare reimbursement rates in Part Four of the Atlas are from the 1993 Continuous Medicare History Sample (CHMS), which documents reimbursements by calendar year for each component of the Medicare program. The data are for a 5% sample of Medicare enrollees selected on the basis of the terminal digits in the Social Security number (05, 20, 45, 70 or 95). The denominator for rates is the corresponding 5% sample of the enrollment file (see Part Nine, Section 3.1).

4.1 Categories of Medicare Reimbursement Examined in Part Four of the Atlas

Categories of Medicare reimbursement in the Atlas are listed in Table 4 with their definitions from the CHMS file.

4.2 Calculation of Adjusted Medicare Program Rates

Adjustments were made for age, sex, and race as described in Section 3.2. Adjustments for differences in price were made using the method described in Section 2.3, with two differences. First, in order to calculate the HRR-level modified GPCI, we used the number of Medicare enrollees in each HRR as the weight, rather than the general population. Second, because Medicare Part B payments compensate for only one-quarter of the difference in professional wage adjustments across areas and include an adjustment for malpractice insurance costs, the same adjustment was made in reverse to recover the original value of Part B billings.

Table 4. Definitions for Categories of Reimbursement in Part Four of the Atlas

Category of Reimbursement	For each service, the specified components were selected from the file and summed as indicated. All fields refer to packed-decimal, variable length, EBCDIC, mainframe record layout locations.
All Services	File: Annual Data trailer Part A Reimb, incl. passthru amts. cols. 14-17 Part B Reimb, incl. passthru amts. cols. 18-21Total Reimb. = Part A + Part B Reimb.
Professional and Laboratory Services	File: Payment trailer 1. Medical line items, cols. 12-13 (TOS=1, 3, Y, Z) 2. Medical Reimb., cols. 17-19 3. Surgical line items, cols. 20-21 (TOS=2, 8) 4. Surgical Reimb., cols. 25-27 5. Lab/X-ray line items, cols. 28-29 (TOS=4, 5) 6. Lab/X-ray Reimb., cols. 33-35 Total Reimb = 2+4+6
Acute Care Hospital Services	File: Short Stay trailer Stays, cols. 4-5 LOS, cols. 8-9 Reimbursement, cols.18-21 Passthru amount, cols. 62-65
Outpatient Hospital Services	Outpatient trailer Total bills, cols. 4-5 Total Reimb., cols. 9-11 Outpatient POS bills, cols. 12-13 Outpatient POS Reimb., cols. 17-19 Inpatient POS bills, cols. 20-21 Inpatient POS bills, cols. 25-27
Home Health Care Services	HHA trailer Part A Reimb., cols. 12-14 Part B Reimb., cols. 23-25 Total Reimb. = Part A + Part B

5. The Physician Workforce Rates

The methods for estimating the per capita rates of physicians serving HSAs and HRRs are analogous to the methods used for estimating the allocation of hospital resources (Section 2). The sources of information on physicians are the American Medical Association (AMA; January 1, 1993) and the American Osteopathic Association (AOA; May 31, 1993) Physician Masterfiles. These files have been used extensively to study physician supply and are the only comprehensive data available on physician location, specialty and level of effort devoted to clinical practice. Both the AMA and the AOA physician files classify physicians according to self-reported level of effort devoted to clinical practice. In this study, we excluded physicians who reported that they worked the majority of the time in medical teaching, administration or research, and part time physicians working fewer than 20 hours a week in clinical practice. Interns, residents and fellows training in specific specialties were not included in the rates for specialists presented in Part Five. Both files also list ZIP Code fields indicating the physician's primary place of practice, which was complete in more than 90% of records. When this information was not available, we used the physician's preferred professional address to indicate location. Based on these criteria, 469,603 physicians resident in the 50 states and District of Columbia constituted the clinically active physician workforce for 1993. There were also 96,887 physicians in residency or fellowship programs.

5.1 Physician Specialties Considered in Part Five of the Atlas

The AMA and AOA physician files include the physician's primary self-designated specialty from a list of 207 specialties. We grouped these into the categories in Table 5.

Table 5. Categories of Clinically Active Physicians in Part Five of the Atlas

Classification of physician specialties and type of utilization used for allocation and age adjustment

Dartmouth Specialty	AMA or AOA Specialty	AMA/AOA Code	Allocation	Age Adjustment
All Physicians	All except Unspecified (Codes US, T)			
Primary Physicians	Adolescent Medicine-GP	AGP	Medical	Family Practice
	Family Practice	FP		
	Geriatrics Medicine (Family Practice)	FPG		
		FSM		
	General Practice	GP		
	Sports Medicine-GP	SGP		
	Internal Medicine-Emergency Medicine	IEM	Medical	Internal Medicine
	Internal Medicine	IM		
	Internal Medicine-Pediatrics	IPD		
	Pediatrics	PD	Medical	Pediatrics
Specialty Physicians	All except Primary Physicians and Unspecified (Codes US, T)			
Anesthesiology	Anesthesiology	AN	Surgical	Surgery
	Cardiothoracic Anesthesiology	CAN		
	Obstetrics Anesthesiology	OBA		
	Pediatric Anesthesiology	PAN		
Cardiology	Cardiology	C	Medical	Cardiology
	Cardiovascular Diseases	CD		
		CVD		
	Cardiac Electrophysiology	ICE		
General Surgery	Abdominal Surgery	AS	Surgical	General Surgery
	Colon and Rectal Surgery	CRS		
	General Surgery	GS		
	Surgery-General	S		
Obstetrics/ Gynecology	Gynecological Oncology	GO	Surgical	Ob/Gyn
	Gynecological Surgery	GS		
	Gynecology	GYN		
	Maternal & Fetal Medicine	MFM		
	Obstetrics & Gynecology	OBG		
	Obstetrics	OBS		
	Obstetrics/Gynecology Surgery	OGS		
	Reproductive Endocrinology	RE		
	Reproductive Endocrinology	REN		
Ophthalmology	Ophthalmology	OPH	Surgical	Ophthalmology

Dartmouth Specialty	AMA or AOA Specialty	AMA/AOA Code	Allocation	Age Adjustment
Orthopedic Surgery	Hand Surgery (Ortho Surgery)	HSO	Surgical	Orthopedic Surg
	Adult Reconstructive Orthopedics	OAR		
	Pediatric Orthopedics	OP		
	Orthopedics	OR		
	Orthopedic Surgery	ORS		
	Sports Medicine (Orthopedic Surgery)	OSM		
	Orthopedic Surgery - Spine	OSS		
	Orthopedic Trauma	OTR		
Psychiatry	Child Psychiatry	CHP	Medical	Psychiatry
	Psychiatry	P		
	Pediatric Psychiatry	PDP		
	Psychoanalysis	PYA		
	Geriatric Psychiatry	PYG		
	Psychosomatic Medicine	PYM		
Radiology	Angiography/Interventional Radiology	ANG	All	not age adjusted
	Diagnostic Radiology	DR		
	Diagnostic Ultrasound	DUS		
	Nuclear Medicine	NM		
	Nuclear Radiology	NR		
	Neuroradiology	NRA		
	Pediatric Radiology	PDR		
	Radiology	R		
	Diagnostic Roentgenology	RTD		
Urology	Urological Surgery	U	Surgical	Urology
	Urology	URS		

5.2 Allocation of Clinically Active Physicians

Clinically active physicians were assigned to the HSAs of their primary place of practice or preferred professional address. Since physicians, like hospitals, provide services to patients residing outside of the HSA in which their practices are located, the physician workforce was allocated to adjust for patient migration. Unfortunately, allocations could not be based on information about the travel patterns of the patients of individual physicians or information about the use of care outside acute hospitals. For clinically active non-federal physicians (N=456,030), the adjustments are closely analogous to the method used for hospital resources, with an important exception. Since the hospital affiliations of the physicians was not determined, the physicians were allocated on the basis of the patterns of inpatient care of all the hospitals located in their HSAs. The MEDPAR records selected for allocation, which depended on the physician's specialty, are given in Table 5. For example, primary physicians were allocated on the basis of medical DRGs. If an HSA had 4 primary care physicians and if 25% of the medical DRG patient days at the local hospital(s) in 1992-93 were for residents of a neighboring HSA, then the four primary physicians would be estimated to contribute 1.0 FTE primary care physician to the neighboring HSA.

We included clinically active federal physicians (N=13,573) in the study, since these physicians serve populations counted by the U.S. census, such as veterans, residents of Indian reservations, medically underserved areas, and military personnel and their dependents. Federal physicians were assigned to either the Department of Defense/ Public Health Service (DoD/PHS) or the Department of Veterans Affairs (VA) in proportion to the mix of staffed federal beds within each HSA (U.S. Medicine; DoD technical document). All federal pediatricians and obstetrician/gynecologists were assigned to the DoD/ PHS. DoD/PHS physicians were allocated to HSAs in the same proportion as the non-federal physicians. Since VA utilization data were available that were analogous to the Medicare Part A data, VA physicians were allocated to areas in proportion to VA inpatient utilization (e.g., if 25% of the patient days of VA hospitals in Manhattan were provided to veterans residing in the Bronx, then 25% of the VA physicians in New York were assigned to the Bronx). If no federal inpatient facility (DoD, VAH, PHS, Indian Health Service) was present within the HSA, then the physicians were assumed to represent primary care and were allocated in the same proportion as non-federal primary care physicians (using inpatient medical days).

When all physician specialty groups had been allocated to HSAs, their allocated FTEs were summed. The primary care physicians allocated to an HSA represent the total of all federal and non-federal FTE physicians allocated from local as well as remote HSAs. For the HSAs in a given HRR, physician resources were further summed to obtain the total for the HRR. Crude rates were then calculated for HRRs using the 1990 population for all ages described in section 1.4.

Measures of physicians in residency training programs presented in the Atlas were prepared using similar methods.

5.3 Calculation of Adjusted Rates

The allocation rates presented in Part Five of the Atlas were adjusted for age and sex using the indirect method. Since age-sex specific physician utilization rates by specialty are not available for all medical care services, we used outpatient age, sex and specialty specific physician visit rates from the combined 1989-1992 National Ambulatory Care Survey (NAMCS) as the standard. NAMCS specialty categories matched the AMA and AOA categories. Three specialties could not be age and sex adjusted because of the low frequency of ambulatory visits: critical care, pathology, and radiology.

6. Diagnostic and Surgical Procedure Rates

The rates of inpatient surgery in Part Six are based on the MEDPAR files for 1992 and 1993. To insure that the population included in the numerator corresponded to the denominator population, restrictions were applied to exclude the following records: Medicare enrollees under age 65 or over age 99 on June 30, 1992 or 1993; Medicare enrollees in risk-bearing HMOs; MEDPAR records with a length of stay over 365 days; and hospitalizations at psychiatric, rehabilitation or long term care units (provider codes = S, T, U or V; facility type not equal to S; third digit of Medicare provider number not equal to 0). The rates of diagnostic procedures are based on a 5% sample of the 1993 Physician (Part B) Claims file. The denominators are the 1992-93 Medicare enrollee population and the 5% 1993 Medicare enrollee population described in Section 1.4, respectively.

6.1 Procedures examined in Part Six of the Atlas

The procedure codes used in Part Six are listed in Table 6. The procedure codes used in the MEDPAR file are based on the International Classification of Disease, ICD-9-CM. For diagnostic procedures, the Current Procedure Terminology convention was used. Selection of procedure codes was based on review of the literature and/or consultation with clinical experts. No rate was based on a count of fewer than 15 events.

6.2 Calculation of Adjusted Procedure-Specific Rates

Indirect-adjusted rates were computed as described in Section 3.2. All rates were adjusted for age, sex, and race, except that sex-specific population estimates were used for prostate and breast procedures. Rates were age and race adjusted as described above (3.2).

Table 6. Definitions of Procedures and Conditions

Condition	Source File	Codes used to define condition
Coronary Artery Disease		
Coronary artery bypass surgery	MEDPAR	Procedure code (any position) 36.10 - 36.19
PTCA	MEDPAR	Procedure code (any position) 36.01, 36.02, 36.05
Coronary angiography	Part A	CPT code 93547 - 93553
Breast Cancer (f)		
Mammography	Part B	CPT code 76090 - 76092
Partial mastectomy	MEDPAR	Procedure code (principal position) 85.20 - 85.23*
Simple or radical mastectomy	MEDPAR	Procedure code 85.41, 85.43, 85.45, 85.47* (*must have diagnosis code 174 as well)
Treatment of Back Pain		
Laminectomy, spinal fusion	MEDPAR	Procedure code 03.09, 80.5 - 80.59, 81.0 - 81.09
Early Prostate Cancer (m)		
Needle biopsy	Part B	CPT 55700
Radical prostatectomy	MEDPAR	Procedure code 60.5
Benign Prostatic Hyperplasia (BPH) (m)		
Transurethral resection for BPH	MEDPAR	Procedure code 60.2, 60.20 and Diagnosis codes 600-601.4, 601.8, 601.9, 602-602.1, 602.3, 602.8, 602.9, or 788.2

Note: (f) refers to procedures for which counts of women served as the denominator; (m) refers to procedures for which counts of men served as the denominator

7. Benchmarking

The variations in per capita resource allocations and utilization among HRRs provide the basis for asking "What if?" questions. For example, if the numbers of hospital beds per 1,000 residents in a particular HRR were the standard for the United States, how many more or how many fewer beds would be required? Or, if the numbers of primary care physicians per 100,000 residents observed for another HRR were the standard for your HRR, how many more or how many fewer primary physicians would be needed?

Part Seven of the Atlas provides examples of how benchmarking can be applied to answer such questions. For example, the physician supply in the United States was compared to the physician workforce employed in a large staff model HMO and the Minneapolis HRR. The HMO physician rates were obtained from an ongoing study of HMO physician workforce market dynamics sponsored by the Robert Wood Johnson Foundation (personal communication, David Kindig, M.D., University of Wisconsin). The study protocols were designed to take out-of-plan use into account in estimating the per capita size of the workforce. In calculating the HMO rate for primary physicians, we included emergency physicians because this specialty provided much of the acute and after-hours primary care in the HMO. The HMO workforce rates, like the rates for HRRs, were age and sex adjusted to the U.S. population as described in Section 5.3. Thus, the rates can be compared without concern that differences in age and sex structure might explain the observed differences.

The strategies for benchmarking used in Part Seven permit comparisons of age and sex adjusted rates across areas and provide estimates of the numbers of physicians in excess or in deficit of the benchmark health plan or HRR. The rates referenced in Table Two, Part Eight provide the data from which the information in Figure 7.1 – the supply of physicians in the United States benchmarked to a large HMO – was derived. For example, the ratio of U.S. rates for orthopedic surgeons (7.2 per 100,000 residents) to the HMO employment pattern (4.5 per 100,000 enrollees) is 1.60, indicating a 60% surplus in the national supply, if the HMO was used as the benchmark. According to this benchmark, the number of orthopedic physicians in the U.S. in excess of "need" is obtained by evaluating:

(U.S. rate-HMO rate) x (U.S Population/100,000) = (7.2 - 4.5) x (2,486.5) = 6,706 physicians

Figure 7.3 benchmarks the experience of the HMO to a single city, Minneapolis. For example, the ratio of Minneapolis rates for radiologists (7.52 per 100,000) compared to the HMO employment pattern (8.70 per 100,000) is 0.86, indicating a 14% deficit in the Minneapolis supply, compared to the HMO employment rate. According to the HMO benchmark, the number of radiologists serving the Minneapolis HRR is in undersupply:

(Minneapolis rate - HMO rate) x (Minneapolis Population/100,000) = (7.52-8.70) x (26.1) =
-30.8 FTE Radiologists

The data in the tables in Part Eight are adjusted to the U.S. population and can be used to benchmark the experience in your own region to the region of your choice. Find the rate in your own area for the resource allocation, hospitalization or procedure rate of interest. Then identify the benchmark region to which you wish to make the comparison. The ratio of the experience in your region to the benchmark is obtained by dividing your rate by the rate in the benchmark region. The numbers of hospital beds, personnel, expenditures, physicians, hospitalizations, or diagnostic or surgical procedures above or below the benchmark is obtained by the following formula:

(your HRR rate - benchmark rate) x (your HRR population/rate convention) = excess (+) or deficit
(-) in resources, hospitalizations, procedures, according to the selected benchmark

The "rate convention," i.e., the denomination used for calculating population rates in the tables presented in Part Eight, is: for expenditures and reimbursements, per person; for procedures, hospitalizations and hospital beds and personnel, per 1,000; for physician workforce, per 100,000.

Please note that data benchmarked using Medicare procedure rates per thousand residents are for a two-year period, 1992-93; the appropriate population is the two-year person-year estimate given in Table Three in Part Eight. For readability, the rates in Tables One through Four have been rounded, usually to one place to the right of the decimal point. Data displayed in the maps and in the figures in Parts One through Eight are fully precise. As a result, calculations of the numbers in the benchmark figures starting from the rounded numbers in the tables yield approximate, but not exactly the same, estimates. Despite the rounding, the precision in the tables is sufficient for making comparisons between regions. The machine-readable data base available with the Atlas can be used to achieve full precision.

Map List

Map	Title	Table	Displayed Data Variable Name
1.1	ZIP Codes Assigned to the Windsor, Vermont Hospital Service Area		
1.2	Hospital Service Areas According to the Number of Acute Care Hospitals		
1.3	Hospital Service Areas According to Population Size		
1.4	Hospital Service Areas Assigned to the Evansville, Indiana Hospital Referral Region		
1.5	Hospital Referral Regions According to the Number of Hospitals Performing Major Cardiovascular Surgery		
1.6	New England Hospital Referral Regions		
1.7	Northeast Hospital Referral Regions		
1.8	South Atlantic Hospital Referral Regions		
1.9	Southeast Hospital Referral Regions		
1.10	South Central Hospital Referral Regions		
1.11	Southwest Hospital Referral Regions		
1.12	Great Lakes Hospital Referral Regions		
1.13	Upper Midwest Hospital Referral Regions		
1.14	Rocky Mountain Hospital Referral Regions		
1.15	Pacific Northwest Hospital Referral Regions		
1.16	Pacific Coast Hospital Referral Regions		
2.1	Acute Care Hospital Beds	1	Adjusted Beds per 1000
2.2	Acute Care Hospital Employees	1	Adjusted FTE per 1000
2.3	Registered Nurses Employed in Acute Care Hospitals	1	Adjusted RNs per 1000
2.4	Total Acute Care Hospital Expenditures	1	Adjusted Total Expenditures per Capita
4.1	Price Adjusted Medicare Reimbursements for Traditional (Noncapitated) Medicare	4	Price Adjusted Total A and B Reimbursements
4.2	Price Adjusted Medicare Reimbursements for Professional and Laboratory Services	4	Price Adjusted Part B Professional and Lab Services
4.3	Price Adjusted Medicare Reimbursements for Inpatient Hospital Services	4	Price Adjusted Part A Short Stay Reimbursements
4.4	Price Adjusted Medicare Reimbursements for Outpatient Facilities	4	Price Adjusted Outpatient Facilities Reimbursements
4.5	Price Adjusted Medicare Reimbursements for Home Health Care Services	4	Price Adjusted Home Health Reimbursements
4.6	Medicare Enrollment in Capitated Managed Care Plans		
4.7	Variations in Medicare Reimbursements		
5.1	The Physician Workforce Active in Patient Care	2	All Physicians

Map	Title	Table	Displayed Data Variable Name
5.2	Physicians in Primary Care	2	Primary Care Physicians
5.3	Specialist Physicians	2	Specialists
5.a	The 50/50 Rule		
5.4	Anesthesiologists	2	Anesthesiologists
5.5	Cardiologists	2	Cardiologists
5.6	General Surgeons	2	General Surgeons
5.7	Obstetrician/Gynecologists	2	Obstetrician/Gynecologists
5.8	Ophthalmologists	2	Ophthalmologists
5.9	Orthopedic Surgeons	2	Orthopedic Surgeons
5.10	Psychiatrists	2	Psychiatrists
5.11	Radiologists	2	Radiologists
5.12	Urologists	2	Urologists
5.13	Physicians in Residency Training Programs	2	Resident Physicians
6.1	Coronary Artery Bypass Grafting	3	CABG Procedure Rate
6.2	Percutaneous Transluminal Coronary Angioplasty	3	PTCA Procedure Rate
6.3	Coronary Angiography	3	Part A Angiography Rate
6.4	Mammography	3	Part B Mammography Incidence Rate
6.5	Breast Sparing Surgery	3	Part A Percent Partial Mastectomies
6.6	Back Surgery	3	Back Surgery Rate
6.7	Prostate Biopsy	3	Part B Prostate Biopsy Incidence Rate
6.8	Radical Prostatectomy	3	Radical Prostatectomy Rate
6.9	Transurethral Resection of the Prostate	3	TURP and BPH Rate

Figure List

Figure	Title	Table	Ordinate Variable Name	Table	Abscissa Variable Name	R²
3.8	The Association Between Allocated Hospital Beds and Population Based Medicare Mortality	3	Medicare Mortality Rate	1	Adjusted Beds per 1000	.13
3.9	The Association Between Hospital Capacity and Medicare Hospitalization Rates for High Variation Medical Conditions Among Populations, Stratified by Median Income in ZIP Code of Residence		Breakdown of High Variation Medical Conditions by Income is not in the Tables			
4.1	Price Adjusted Reimbursements for Traditional (Noncapitated) Medicare Among Hospital Referral Regions (1993)	4	Dartmouth Price Adjusted Total A and B Reimbursements			
4.2	Price Adjusted Part B Medicare Reimbursements for Professional and Laboratory Services Among Hospital Referral Regions (1993)	4	HCFA Price Adjusted Part B Professional and Lab Services			
4.3	Price Adjusted Reimbursements for Inpatient Hospital Services Among Hospital Referral Regions (1993)	4	Dartmouth Price Adjusted Part A Short Stay Reimbursements			
4.4	Price Adjusted Medicare Reimbursements for Outpatient Services Among Hospital Referral Regions (1993)	4	Dartmouth Price Adjusted Outpatient Facilities Reimbursements			
4.5	Price Adjusted Medicare Reimbursements for Home Health Care Services Among Hospital Referral Regions (1993)	4	Dartmouth Price Adjusted Home Health Care Reimbursements			
4.6	The Association Between Price Adjusted Medicare Reimbursements for Outpatient and Inpatient Hospital Services (1993)	4	Dartmouth Price Adjusted Part A Short Stay Reimbursements	4	Dartmouth Price Adjusted Outpatient Facilities Reimbursements	.17
4.7	The Association Between Price Adjusted Medicare Reimbursements for Professional and Laboratory Services and for Inpatient Hospital Services (1993)	4	Dartmouth Price Adjusted Part A Short Stay Reimbursements	4	HCFA Price Adjusted Part B Professional and Lab Services	.23
4.8	The Association Between Price Adjusted Medicare Part B Reimbursements Provided Outside and Inside the Hospital (1993)		Physician Inpatient Services not included in the Tables		Physician Services not included in the Tables	.52
5.1	Physicians Allocated to Hospital Referral Regions (1993)	2	All Physicians			
5.2	Primary Care Physicians Allocated to Hospital Referral Regions (1993)	2	Primary Care Physicians			
5.3	Specialists Allocated to Hospital Referral Regions (1993)	2	Specialists			
5.a	The Association Between the Specialty Physician Workforce and Price Adjusted Medicare Medical and Surgical Reimbursements (1993)	4	HCFA Price Adjusted Part B Medical and Surgical Services	2	Specialists	.15
5.b	The Association Between the Primary Care Physician Workforce and Price Adjusted Medicare Medical and Surgical Reimbursements (1993)	4	HCFA Price Adjusted Part B Medical and Surgical Services	2	Primary Care Physicians	.01
5.4	Anesthesiologists Allocated to Hospital Referral Regions (1993)	2	Anesthesiologists			

Figure	Title	Table	Ordinate Variable Name	Table	Abscissa Variable Name	R²
7.2	Ratios of the Rates of Supply of Physicians in the United States to Rates in the Minneapolis Hospital Referral Region (1993)				Observed Physician Rates	
					Expected Physician Rates	
					Observed to Expected Ratio for Physicians	
7.3	Ratios of the Rates of Supply of Physicians in Minneapolis to Rates in a Large Health Maintenance Organization (1993)				Observed Physician Rates	
					Expected Physician Rates	
					Observed to Expected Ratio for Physicians	
7.4	Ratios of the Rates for Medicare Reimbursements and for Hospital Resource Allocations in the United States to the Rates in the Minneapolis Hospital Referral Region (1993)			4	Total Part A and Part B Reimbursements	
				4	Outpatient Facilities Reimbursements	
				4	Part A Short Stay Reimbursements	
				4	Part B Reimbursements for Professional and Lab Services	
				4	Home Health Care Reimbursements	
				1	Adjusted Beds per 1000	
				1	Adjusted FTE per 1000	
				1	Adjusted RNs per 1000	
7.5	Ratios of the Rates of Physicians in Selected HRRs to Rates in the Minneapolis Hospital Referral Region (1993)				Observed Physician Rates	
					Expected Physician Rates	
					Observed to Expected Ratio for Physicians	
7.6	Ratios of the Rates for Hospital Resources and Medicare Reimbursement in Selected HRRs to Rates in the Minneapolis Hospital Referral Region (1993)			1	Adjusted Beds per 1000	
				1	Adjusted FTE per 1000	
				1	Adjusted RNs per 1000	
				4	Total Part A and Part B Reimbursements	

The Dartmouth Atlas of Health Care is based, in part, on data supplied by
The American Hospital Association
The American Medical Association
The American Osteopathic Association
The Health Care Financing Administration
The National Center for Health Statistics
The United States Census
The United States Department of Defense
Claritas, Incorporated

Data analyses were performed using
Software developed by the Center for the Evaluative Clinical Sciences
using SAS® on HP® equipment running the UNIX® system software

Maps and map databases were generated using
MapInfo® software
Highway map coordinates from MapInfo®
ZIP Code map coordinates from GDT®
Claritas 3H. Custom Dataset for US ZIP Codes from Claritas®

Atlas design and print production by

Elizabeth Adams and Jonathan Sa'adah
Intermedia Print Communications, Hartford, Vermont